CLINICAL MANAGEMENT OF RIGHT HEMISPHERE DYSFUNCTION

SECOND EDITION

THE REHABILITATION INSTITUTE OF CHICAGO PUBLICATION SERIES
Don A. Olson, PhD, Series Coordinator

Spinal Cord Injury: A Guide to Functional Outcomes in Physical Therapy Management

Lower Extremity Amputation: A Guide to Functional Outcomes in Physical Therapy Management, Second Edition

Stroke/Head Injury: A Guide to Functional Outcomes in Physical Therapy Management

Clinical Evaluation of Dysphagia

Spinal Cord Injury: A Guide to Functional Outcomes in Occupational Therapy

Spinal Cord Injury: A Guide to Rehabilitation Nursing

Head Injury: A Guide to Functional Outcomes in Occupational Therapy Management

Speech/Language Treatment of the Aphasias: Treatment Materials for Auditory Comprehension and Reading Comprehension

Speech/Language Treatment of the Aphasias: Treatment Materials for Oral Expression and Written Expression

Rehabilitation Nursing Procedures Manual

Psychological Management of Traumatic Brain Injuries in Children and Adolescents

Medical Management of Long-Term Disability

Psychological Aspects of Geriatric Rehabilitation

Clinical Management of Dysphagia in Adults and Children, Second Edition

Spinal Cord Injury: Medical Management and Rehabilitation

Clinical Management of Right Hemisphere Dysfunction, Second Edition

Clinical Management of Communication Problems in Adults with Traumatic Brain Injury

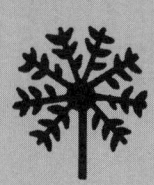

Rehabilitation Institute of Chicago
PROCEDURE MANUAL

CLINICAL MANAGEMENT OF RIGHT HEMISPHERE DYSFUNCTION

SECOND EDITION

Anita S. Halper, MA, CCC-SLP
Reengineering Project Specialist, Rehabilitation Institute of Chicago
Associate Professor, Physical Medicine and Rehabilitation
Northwestern University Medical School
Chicago, Illinois
Clinical Associate Professor, Communication Sciences and Disorders
Northwestern University
Evanston, Illinois

Leora Reiff Cherney, PhD, CCC-SLP
Clinical Researcher, Communicative Disorders
Rehabilitation Institute of Chicago
Assistant Professor, Physical Medicine and Rehabilitation
Northwestern University Medical School
Chicago, Illinois

Martha S. Burns, PhD, CCC-SLP
Adjunct Associate Professor, Speech and Hearing Science
University of Illinois, Champaign-Urbana
Champaign-Urbana, Illinois
Associate Professional Staff, Evanston Hospital
Evanston, Illinois

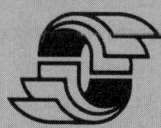

AN ASPEN PUBLICATION®
Aspen Publishers, Inc.
Gaithersburg, Maryland
1996

Library of Congress Cataloging-in-Publication Data
Halper, Anita S.
Clinical management of right hemisphere dysfunction.—2nd ed. /
Anita S. Halper, Leora Reiff Cherney, Martha S. Burns.
p.   cm.—(Rehabilitation Institute of Chicago procedure manual)
Burns' name appears first on earlier edition.
Includes bibliographical references and index.
ISBN 0-8342-0810-5
1. Communicative disorders. 2. Brain damage—Complications.
3. Cognition disorders. 4. Cerebral dominance.
5. Brain—Localization of functions. I. Cherney, Leora Reiff.
II. Burns, Martha S. III. Title. IV. Series.
[DNLM: 1. Dominance, Cerebral. 2. Brain Damage, Chronic—therapy.
3. Brain Damage, Chronic—complications. 4. Communicative
Disorders—etiology.
WL 335 H195c 1996]
RC423.B86 1996
616.8—dc20
DNLM/DLC
for Library of Congress
96-2715
CIP

Copyright © 1996 by Aspen Publishers, Inc.
All rights reserved.

Aspen Publishers, Inc., grants permission for photocopying for limited personal or internal use. This consent does not extend to other kinds of copying, such as copying for general distribution, for advertising or promotional purposes, for creating new collective works, or for resale. For information, address Aspen Publishers, Inc., Permissions Department, 200 Orchard Ridge Drive, Suite 200, Gaithersburg, Maryland 20878.

The authors have made every effort to ensure the accuracy of the information herein, particularly with regard to technique and procedure. However, appropriate information sources should be consulted, especially for new or unfamiliar procedures. It is the responsibility of every practitioner to evaluate the appropriateness of a particular opinion in the context of actual clinical situations and with due consideration to new developments. Authors, editors, and the publisher cannot be held responsible for any typographical or other errors found in this book.

Orders: (800) 638-8437
Customer Service: (800) 234-1660

About Aspen Publishers • For more than 35 years, Aspen has been a leading professional publisher in a variety of disciplines. Aspen's vast information resources are available in both print and electronic formats. We are committed to providing the highest quality information available in the most appropriate format for our customers. Visit Aspen's Internet site for more information resources, directories, articles, and a searchable version of Aspen's full catalog, including the most recent publications:
http://www.aspenpub.com
Aspen Publishers, Inc. • The hallmark of quality in publishing
Members of the worldwide Wolters Kluwer group

Editorial Resources: Jane Colilla
Library of Congress Catalog Card Number: 96-2715
ISBN: 0-8342-0810-5

Printed in the United States of America

1 2 3 4 5

*We would like to extend
a special note of thanks to
Don A. Olson, PhD,
Director, Education and Training,
Rehabilitation Institute of Chicago,
for his continued support of
our professional endeavors.*

Table of Contents

Contributors ix

Preface xi

Chapter 1—Hemispheric Specialization: A History of Current Concepts 1
Martha S. Burns and Jeffrey L. Cummings

    Introduction 1
    Paul Broca and the Dominance of the Left Hemisphere 1
    Disconnection Syndromes and the Split Brain 2
    Modular Theory and Cerebral Networks in Cognitive Processing 4
    Hemispheric Specialization and the Functions of the Right Cerebral
        Hemisphere 4
    The Search for Organizational Principles 7

Chapter 2—Neurological Syndromes Associated with Right Hemisphere Damage 9
Jeffrey L. Cummings and Martha S. Burns

    Introduction 9
    Anatomical and Biochemical Differences Between the Hemispheres 9
    Clinical Syndromes Associated with Right Hemisphere Lesions 11
    Comment 17

**Chapter 3—A Conceptual Framework for the Evaluation and Treatment of
        Communication Problems Associated with Right Hemisphere Damage** 21
Leora Reiff Cherney and Anita S. Halper

    Introduction 21
    Cognitive Processes 23

    Effective Communication Skills 26
    Interrelationships Among the Processes 27
    Conclusion 27

Chapter 4— RIC Evaluation of Communication Problems in Right Hemisphere Dysfunction-Revised (RICE-R): Statistical Background 31
Leora Reiff Cherney, Anita S. Halper, Allen W. Heinemann, and Patrick Semik

    Introduction 31
    Phase 1: Establishing Internal Consistency of the Items 32
    Phase 2: Standardization of the RICE-R 33
    Conclusion 40

Chapter 5— Tests for Evaluating Cognitive-Communicative Skills in Patients with Right Hemisphere Damage 41
Anita S. Halper and Leora Reiff Cherney

Chapter 6— Treatment of Cognitive-Communicative Skills in Patients with Right Hemisphere Damage 57
Anita S. Halper, Leora Reiff Cherney, and Martha S. Burns

    Introduction 57
    Attention 59
    Perception 67
    Memory 72
    Orientation 79
    Pragmatics 81
    Higher-Level Cognitive Processes (Organization, Reasoning, and Problem Solving or Judgment) 89
    Appendix 6–A: Guidelines for Communication Management: Family and Staff ... 97
    Appendix 6–B: Publishers of Treatment Materials and Computer Programs 98

Appendix A—RIC Evaluation of Communication Problems in Right Hemisphere Dysfunction-Revised (RICE-R) 99
Anita S. Halper, Leora Reiff Cherney, Martha S. Burns, and Shelley I. Mogil

Appendix B— RIC Evaluation of Communication Problems in Right Hemisphere Dysfunction-Revised (RICE-R)—Administration Manual 117
Anita S. Halper, Leora Reiff Cherney, Martha S. Burns, and Shelley I. Mogil

Index 133

Contributors

Martha S. Burns, PhD, CCC-SLP
Adjunct Associate Professor
Speech and Hearing Science
University of Illinois, Champaign-Urbana
Champaign-Urbana, Illinois
Associate Professional Staff
Evanston Hospital
Evanston, Illinois

Leora Reiff Cherney, PhD, CCC-SLP
Clinical Researcher: Communicative Disorders
Rehabilitation Institute of Chicago
Assistant Professor
Physical Medicine and Rehabilitation
Northwestern University Medical School
Chicago, Illinois

Jeffrey L. Cummings, MD
Professor
Neurology and Psychiatry
University of California, Los Angeles
Los Angeles, California

Anita S. Halper, MA, CCC-SLP
Reengineering Project Specialist
Rehabilitation Institute of Chicago
Associate Professor
Physical Medicine and Rehabilitation
Northwestern University Medical School
Chicago, Illinois
Clinical Associate Professor
Communication Sciences and Disorders
Northwestern University
Evanston, Illinois

Allen W. Heinemann, PhD
Director
Rehabilitation Services Evaluation Unit
Rehabilitation Institute of Chicago
Associate Professor
Physical Medicine and Rehabilitation
Northwestern University Medical School
Chicago, Illinois

Shelley I. Mogil, MS, MM, CCC-SP
Associate
Rosalind Reed Associates
Oak Park, Illinois

Patrick Semik, BA
Data Manager
Department of Research
Rehabilitation Institute of Chicago
Chicago, Illinois

Preface

In 1985, the first edition of *Clinical Management of Right Hemisphere Dysfunction* was published. At that time, attention to the function of the right hemisphere was increasing and professionals in a variety of fields were expanding their efforts to better understand the constellation of cognitive-communicative disturbances that affect this population. The goal of this first edition had been to provide a comprehensive yet practical compendium for effective management of these patients.

This second edition provides updated information on hemispheric specialization, including a discussion of modular theory and cerebral networks in cognitive processing with implications for the role of the right hemisphere. In addition, a schematic representation of the relationships among different cognitive processes is presented to serve as a clinical guide for evaluation and treatment. The RIC Evaluation of Communication Problems in Right Hemisphere Dysfunction (RICE) that was presented in the 1985 edition has been revised and has undergone a standardization process. The revised test, an administration manual, and data for interpretation of test results are provided. Finally, treatment objectives, procedures, and measures that are consistent with current trends in health care are presented.

In Chapter 1, Burns and Cummings summarize the current understanding of hemispheric specialization and the role of the right hemisphere. In Chapter 2, Cummings and Burns present the anatomical and biochemical differences between the two hemispheres as well as the clinical syndromes resulting from unilateral right hemisphere damage.

In Chapter 3, Cherney and Halper present a conceptual framework for the clinical management of cognitive-communicative impairments associated with right hemisphere damage. In Chapter 4, The RIC Evaluation of Communication Problems in Right Hemisphere Dysfunction-Revised (RICE-R) is discussed. Cherney, Halper, Heinemann, and Semik address the development of the RICE-R and provide data on the reliability and validity of the test collected as part of the standardization process. The RICE-R test and the administration manual are presented in appendixes at the end of the book. These forms may be reproduced for clinical use. An annotated list of formal standardized tests that are useful for assessing cognitive-communicative skills in patients with right hemisphere damage has been compiled by Halper and Cherney and is presented in Chapter 5. In Chapter 6, Halper, Cherney, and Burns focus on treatment objectives and procedures for patients with right hemisphere damage.

It is our hope that rehabilitation clinicians will find this book helpful in daily clinical practice and a welcome addition to their library.

Chapter 1

Hemispheric Specialization: A History of Current Concepts

Martha S. Burns and Jeffrey L. Cummings

INTRODUCTION

Development of the current understanding of hemispheric specialization can be divided into four historical eras. The first era concerned the discovery of dominance of the left hemisphere for language. Paul Broca was a principal figure in this initial discovery. The second era involved explaining the role of the white matter tracts that connect areas within the same hemisphere and that provide connections between the two hemispheres. The major contributors in this period were Roger Sperry and Norman Geschwind. During the third era there was a rapid expansion of knowledge regarding the functions of the right hemisphere. This period restored a balanced view of the roles of each of the hemispheres, emphasizing that both hemispheres make distinctive contributions to the ecology of human intelligence. The fourth era has emphasized local neural circuits involved in different aspects of human cognitive processing. Whereas studies of the left versus right hemisphere in the third era stressed a horizontal dichotomy across the two hemispheres, studies of neural circuits in the most recent era have uncovered cognitive pathways that connect cortical and subcortical structures. Some of these circuits originate in limbic and subcortical regions with way stations for information processing at various cerebral regions. In many cases, these vertical circuits seem to involve primarily one hemisphere or the other, depending upon the cognitive demands of the task. Thus, the fourth era has broadened our understanding of the ways in which one hemisphere might preferentially mediate one type of processing compared to another.

This history represents an evolution of understanding of the roles of the two hemispheres, with each period revising and adding information. To a great extent, our understanding has unfolded as a direct result of improved neuroimaging technology. New and improved neuroimaging techniques continue to clarify our window into the working human brain. This chapter reviews the historical periods in the evolution of the knowledge of hemisphere specialization and provides an overview of the functions of the two hemispheres.

PAUL BROCA AND THE DOMINANCE OF THE LEFT HEMISPHERE

Broca's discovery of the dominance of the left hemisphere for language was anticipated by localizationist theories that were proffered early in the

19th century. The most well known of these early concepts were promulgated by Franz Joseph Gall and his student Johann Gaspar Spurzheim, who fostered a school of thought known as *phrenology* and maintained that mental functions could be localized in the brain. They further contended that the relative development of mental functions resulted in deformations of the overlying skull such that an individual's abilities could be determined simply by palpating the shape of the cranium.[1] The latter idea enjoyed great popularity among the lay public but was ridiculed by the scientific community and gradually lost favor in the early 1800s. Although Gall was an accomplished anatomist and his ideas presaged many contemporary concepts of hemispheric specialization, his association with phrenology led others to link the concepts together and to deprecate theories of cerebral localization.

After Gall's death in 1828, J.B. Bouillaud, among others, continued to champion the concept of functional localization within the hemispheres, but major and enduring support for an association between localized brain regions and specific neuropsychological activities came only with the discoveries of Paul Broca.[2,3] In 1861, Broca, a French physician and anthropologist, reported two cases of aphasia associated with left-sided frontal lobe lesions. Two years later, he described the autopsy results of eight patients with aphasia and noted that all lesions involved the third frontal convolution on the left.[4,5] This momentous observation provided the basis for all future investigation of hemispheric specialization. Broca appeared to have realized the profundity of his discovery when he stated: "And, a most remarkable thing, in all of these patients the lesion existed on the left side. I do not dare to draw a conclusion and I await new facts."[4] Confirmatory findings were not long in coming, and a special role for the left hemisphere in mediating language function was soon firmly established.

Carl Wernicke made the next important observation regarding the dominance of the left hemisphere for linguistic abilities. At the age of 26, Wernicke published a small monograph on aphasia in which he described sensory aphasia for the first time and discussed the importance of the fibers connecting the posterior temporal with the inferior frontal regions of the left hemisphere.[1] In addition to refining understanding of the role of the left cerebral hemisphere in the mediation of language, Wernicke's discoveries contributed to the growing impression that the left hemisphere was dominant for many and perhaps most intellectual functions.

This belief in the general dominance of the left hemisphere was further encouraged by Hugo Liepmann, who published his papers describing the apraxias in 1900.[1] Liepmann observed that apraxia was more common with left-sided rather than right-sided lesions, thus providing support for the major role of the left hemisphere in certain motor activities as well as in language function.

Despite occasional observations to the contrary, the view of the left cerebral hemisphere as dominant for most intellectual functions was endorsed from the late 19th century to the mid-20th century. Indeed, animals were thought to have the equivalent of two right hemispheres, and human phylogenetic supremacy was attributed solely to the accomplishments made possible by the dominant left hemisphere.[6] This lopsided view of cerebral function was challenged by descriptions of behavioral deficits following focal right-sided damage, but major advances in reforming the concepts of a general left hemisphere dominance awaited discoveries concerning the role of white matter tracts in providing intrahemispheric and interhemispheric connections.

DISCONNECTION SYNDROMES AND THE SPLIT BRAIN

The role of the corpus callosum and the white matter of the brain had long been an enigma. Galen, in the second century AD, postulated that thoughts were generated in the cerebral ventricles and saw no role for the corpus callosum. In 1664, Thomas Willis suggested that the callosum was the seat of the imagination. Felix Vicq d'Azyr, a French anatomist and personal physician to Marie Antoinette, held the first modern view of the corpus callosum. In 1784, he suggested: "The commissures are intended to establish sympathetic communications between different parts of the brain, just as the nerves do between different organs and the brain itself."[7]

The first clinical syndromes attributed to disruption of the corpus callosum were described by Joseph Jules Dejerine and Hugo Liepmann. Dejerine, in 1892, described a patient who suddenly developed a right homonymous hemianopia along with an inability to read. Paradoxically, the patient retained the capacity to write in spite of the inability to read his own writing. The patient died and at autopsy was found to have a lesion in the left occipital region and the posterior aspect of the corpus callosum. Dejerine postulated that the syndrome reflected the blindness of the right visual field (produced by the left occipital lesion) and an inability to transfer visual information from the intact right hemisphere to the left hemispheric language areas through the damaged corpus callosum.[8] The callosal lesion thus disrupted transfer of information from the right to the left hemisphere and produced the specific clinical syndrome of alexia without agraphia.

As noted previously, Liepmann had an intense interest in the apraxias, and, in 1907, Liepmann and Maas discovered that a lesion of the corpus callosum resulted in an isolated apraxia involving the left arm and leg.[7] The callosal lesion prevented the transfer of impulses from the left to the right hemisphere for control of the left-sided extremities.

Unfortunately, these early insights into the function of the corpus callosum and the syndromes that result from callosal injury were largely ignored, and the role of the callosum in coordinating the activities of the two hemispheres was lost to investigators succeeding Dejerine and Liepmann. Thus, in the 1930s and 1940s, when Akelaitis and colleagues examined patients with partial or complete sections of the callosum performed for control of epileptic seizures, they were unable to identify any persisting deficits.[7] These observations led inevitably to the conclusion that the corpus callosum played no major role in cerebral function.

This view was challenged by experimental observations made by Ronald Myers and Roger Sperry at the University of Chicago. They found that when the optic chiasm of a cat was severed and the animal was trained with one eye patched, intraocular transfer of information occurred, and the cat performed normally when using the untrained eye alone. If both the chiasm and the corpus callosum were sectioned, however, such transfer of information did not occur. The results implied that the corpus callosum was responsible for transferring the visual information from one hemisphere to the other and that surgical sectioning of the callosum disrupts this normal flow of information.[9,10] These experiments prepared the way for the rediscovery of the role of the corpus callosum in humans.

One of the first modern descriptions of deficits resulting from damage to the corpus callosum in a patient was reported by Norman Geschwind and Edith Kaplan in 1964.[11] They studied a patient who suffered an anterior cerebral artery occlusion with infarction of the anterior portion of the corpus callosum. The patient's deficits included aphasic agraphia when writing with the left hand but not with the right, impaired object identification and tactile letter naming with the left hand but not with the right, and apraxia of the left hand but not of the right. Each of these abnormalities reflects the inability to transfer information between the two hemispheres through the damaged corpus callosum. Aphasic agraphia of the left hand results from the inability to transfer linguistic output from the left to the right hemisphere, which controls the left hand. Left hand anomia is similarly a product of the inability to transfer tactile information, while unilateral apraxia is a product of the inability to transfer a motor command. Following these seminal observations, Geschwind[12] described a series of clinical syndromes resulting from interruption of the corpus callosum or of white matter tracts within the hemispheres. His disconnection hypothesis provided an explanation of many clinical observations, as well as a conceptual framework for understanding the role of white matter tracts in integrating cerebral function.

A more complete explanation of the function of the corpus callosum, the deficits after transection of the callosum, and the abilities of the isolated right hemisphere followed the many observations made by Roger Sperry and his students and colleagues at the California Institute of Technology. They investigated epileptic patients submitted to corpus callosectomy by Joseph Bogen and Philip Vogel for control of epilepsy. These "split-brain" studies corroborated and extended the observations of Geschwind[12] and of Geschwind and Kaplan.[11] The most startling and dramatic revelations of these experiments concerned the diversity and sophistication of neuropsychological capabilities of the right hemisphere, the degree of independent mental activity demonstrable in the disconnected right hemisphere, and the differences in cognitive styles exhibited by the left and right hemispheres. The callosal syndrome described by Liepmann and later by Geschwind and Kaplan[11] was confirmed in the commissurotomized patients. In addition, it was shown that the disconnected right hemisphere possessed at least rudimentary skills for auditory and written language comprehension, that it mediated highly developed visuospatial skills, and that it could provide the basis for a sophisticated emotional and mental life previously considered unique to the language-dominant hemisphere. The discoveries resulting from the study of the commissurotomized patients culminated in the award of the Nobel Prize in Medicine to Sperry in 1982.

MODULAR THEORY AND CEREBRAL NETWORKS IN COGNITIVE PROCESSING

During the past two decades, the application of computer technology to imaging of the human brain has revolutionized the understanding of both the anatomy and the physiology of the working brain.[13] The advent of imaging of the living human brain through computed tomography (CT), magnetic resonance imaging (MRI) and MRI with three-dimensional reconstruction has provided high-resolution anatomical images, permitting study of the relationship between the morphology of the human brain and functional asymmetries observed clinically.[14,15] Further, functional neuroimaging of the working brain through positron emission tomography (PET), single photon emission computed tomography (SPECT), and—more recently—functional MRI (FMRI), EEG brain mapping, and biomagnetometry has permitted investigation of cerebral regions that become relatively more active during processing of specific information.[16] The new information gained from these dynamic imaging technologies has permitted both confirmation and revision of our understanding of localization of cognitive function and of functional asymmetry of the cerebral hemispheres. These observations have led to a revised understanding of the way the human brain processes language, memory, self-awareness, mood, affect, emotion, and reasoning. Intermediary processes, so called because they operate between sensory reception of information and planning and execution of motor acts, are now thought to occur through specifically organized pathways of neurons within the brain that form cerebral networks.[17] These networks course through the limbic system and cerebral association areas.

Various networks have been tentatively identified as responsible for different aspects of cognitive processing, many of them lateralized within one hemisphere. Networks associated with the processing of language in the left hemisphere have been studied carefully during the past decade.[17] Right hemisphere networks have more recently come under investigation. One such network, proposed by Antonio Damasio, links the right hemisphere regions thought to be responsible for mapping and integrating signals from the body with limbic areas responsible for feeling and prefrontal regions associated with reason. Damasio has termed this network the *social emotional circuit* and regards it as a conceivable explanation for the apparent right hemisphere dominance for awareness of body integrity and body in space, as well as awareness of emotions and ability to act in an emotionally conditioned manner.[18]

HEMISPHERIC SPECIALIZATION AND THE FUNCTIONS OF THE RIGHT CEREBRAL HEMISPHERE

In 1874, in an essay entitled "On the Nature of the Duality of the Brain," John Hughlings Jackson first proposed that the two cerebral hemispheres had different functional roles.[19] He hypothesized that the left hemisphere was responsible primarily for mediating verbal activity, whereas the right was devoted to object recognition, as well as to images of places and people.[19] This view anticipated many contemporary ideas concerning the respective functions of the two halves of the brain, but they gained little currency until the split-brain observations described above offered new support for their validity.

A list of functions attributable to each cerebral hemisphere is presented in Table 1–1. The list is derived from observations of patients with focal brain damage to the right hemisphere (see Chapter 2), from studies of commissurectomy (split-brain) patients in which the corpus callosum has been surgically severed allowing each hemisphere to be studied independently, and from experimental investigations of normal subjects through neuropsychological laterality studies and PET and SPECT studies of cerebral metabolism during cognitive tasks. Such studies demonstrate that both hemispheres participate in most intellectual activities but make separate contributions to the cognitive process.

The formal properties of language, especially phonological and syntactic processing, are mediated by the left hemisphere, likely because of a left hemisphere superiority for perception of complex auditory temporal sequences. Speech decoding re-

Table 1–1 Principal Functions of the Two Cerebral Hemispheres

Cognitive Process	Left Hemisphere	Right Hemisphere
Auditory processes	Complex temporal perception	Perception of pitch and melody
Auditory language	Formal properties of language, especially phonological and syntactic encoding and decoding Naming	Social properties of language, including receptive and expressive emotional prosody and pragmatics
Visual-tactile processes	Reading comprehension, especially phonetic decoding Reading aloud Writing Sign language	Reading, especially visually picturable nouns and sight words
Constructions	Internal detail	External configuration
Calculation	Arithmetic processing	Spatial arrangement
Memory	Verbal imagery	Visuospatial imagery Working memory (visuospatial scratch pad)
Attention		Spatial distribution of attention Vigilance
Miscellaneous	Praxis	Emotional facial recognition and discrimination Body image and perception of body in space

quires rapid perception of acoustically complex sequences over time, and the left hemisphere seems to be biologically adapted for speech analysis and synthesis. There is evidence that this left hemisphere preference for processing of complex temporal stimuli may be evident in lower vertebrates as well as human adults.[20]

Constructional deficits, although often considered indicative of right hemisphere damage, are present with lesions of either hemisphere.[21] This suggests that both hemispheres make essential contributions to this visuospatial ability. The two hemispheres, however, each aid the constructional process by providing different types of input.[22,23] The right hemisphere appears to be most involved with providing external details and general orientation and the left hemisphere with contributing internal details.

Calculation, like constructional and linguistic abilities, requires the activities of both hemispheres and can be disturbed by lesions of either. Left hemisphere damage results in an impairment of mathematical symbolization and processing, whereas right hemisphere injury produces disturbances of visuospatial organization of the digits.[24]

Each hemisphere also mediates different aspects of memory. The left hemisphere is essential for verbal memory abilities; the right hemisphere is responsible for nonverbal memory skills.[25]

A few abilities appear to be mediated primarily by one or the other hemisphere. Praxis, the ability to perform learned, skilled movements, is dependent on left hemisphere integrity,[26] whereas the right hemisphere is responsible for recognition and matching of facial expressions.[27]

Thus, each cerebral hemisphere is specialized for the accomplishment of specific tasks or specific aspects of functions performed in common with the contralateral cerebral member. The right hemisphere, formerly relegated to an inferior role and considered capable of only an animal-like level of intellectual performance, is now believed to make essential contributions to many intellectual abilities. The dominance of the left hemisphere for many propositional aspects of language is unchallenged, but the right hemisphere is no

Exhibit 1–1 Dichotomies Proposed To Characterize the Functions of the Two Cerebral Hemispheres

Left Hemisphere	Right Hemisphere
• Verbal	• Nonverbal, visuospatial, preverbal
• Linguistic	• Visual or kinesthetic
• Expression	• Perception
• Auditoarticulary	• Retino-ocular
• Symbolic or propositional	• Visual or imaginative
• Propositioning	• Visual imagery
• Executive	• Storage
• Relations	• Correlates
• Logical, analytic	• Holistic, synthetic
• Propositional	• Appositional
• Serial	• Parallel
• Focal, discrete	• Diffuse
• Difference detecting	• Similarity detecting
• Time dependent	• Time independent
• Segmental	• Spatial, global

longer considered the "minor hemisphere" and is known to be dominant for many intellectual functions.

THE SEARCH FOR ORGANIZATIONAL PRINCIPLES

The demonstration that the two hemispheres are performing complementary but different tasks has led to a search for a single dimension, the two poles of which would represent the function of each of the hemispheres. A list of the dichotomies that have been proposed is presented in Exhibit 1–1.[28–30] Most of the dichotomies emphasize the verbal-linguistic-propositional functions of the left hemisphere and the nonverbal-visuospatial-emotional functions of the right hemisphere. Although such dichotomies are true in a general sense, the investigations reviewed previously have shown that the right hemisphere has considerable linguistic abilities and the left hemisphere makes essential contributions to visuospatial functions.

More broadly encompassing dichotomies have been proposed by Bogen,[28] who suggested that the left hemisphere operates in a propositional mode whereas the right hemisphere has appositional characteristics, and Semmes,[31] who hypothesized that the left hemisphere is organized in a more discretely localized manner whereas right hemispheric organization is more diffuse. Each of these approaches identifies important differences between the functions of the left and right hemispheres, but none is sufficiently inclusive to embrace all neuropsychological abilities of each of the hemispheres. Indeed, it seems unlikely that the two hemispheres are precisely complementary. Each hemisphere has unique capacities and functions but acts in concert with the other under normal circumstances, and each produces a unique pattern of deficits and preserved abilities when damaged.

REFERENCES

1. Eggert GH. *Wernicke's Works on Aphasia: A Sourcebook and Review*. The Hague, The Netherlands: Mouton Publishers; 1977.
2. Duffy CJ. The legacy of association cortex. *Neurology*. 1984;34:192–197.
3. Geschwind N. The organization of language and the brain. *Science*. 1970;170:940–944.
4. Joynt RJ, Benton AL. The memoir of Marc Dax on aphasia. *Neurology*. 1964;14:851–854.
5. Schiller F. *Paul Broca*. Los Angeles, Calif: University of California Press; 1979.
6. Smith A. Dominant and nondominant hemispherectomy. In: Kinsbourne M, Smith WL, eds. *Hemispheric Disconnection and Cerebral Function*. Springfield, Ill: Charles C Thomas Publisher; 1974:5–33.
7. Joynt RJ. The corpus callosum: History of thought regarding its function. In: Kinsbourne M, Smith WL, eds. *Hemispheric Disconnection and Cerebral Function*. Springfield, Ill: Charles C Thomas Publishers; 1974:117–125.
8. Benson DF. The third alexia. *Arch Neurol*. 1977;34:327–331.
9. Gazzaniga MS, LeDoux JE. *The Integrated Mind*. New York, NY: Plenum Publishing Corporation; 1978.
10. Sperry RW. Cerebral organization and behavior. *Science*. 1961;133:1749–1757.
11. Geschwind N, Kaplan E. A human cerebral deconnection syndrome. *Neurology*. 1964;12:675–685.
12. Geschwind N. Disconnection syndromes in animals and man. *Brain*. 1965;88:237–294,585–644.
13. Greenberg JO, ed. *Neuroimaging*. New York, NY: McGraw-Hill Publishing Co; 1995.
14. Witelson SF. Neurology of behavior and cognition: Neuroanatomy and functional asymmetry. Presented at Neurology and Cognition, Northwestern University Medical School; December 13, 1994; Chicago, Ill.
15. Damasio AR. Neuroimaging in behavioral neurology. Presented at Neurology and Cognition, Northwestern University Medical School; December 14, 1994; Chicago, Ill.
16. Matthews MK Jr. Neuroimaging and behavioral neurology. In: Greenberg JO, ed. *Neuroimaging*. New York, NY: McGraw-Hill Publishing Co; 1995.
17. Mesulam MM. Association cortex, frontal lobes and limbic system. Presented at Neurology and Cognition, Northwestern University Medical School; December 15, 1994; Chicago, Ill.
18. Damasio AR. *Descartes' Error: Emotion, Reason and the Human Brain*. New York, NY: Grosset/Putnam; 1994.
19. Jackson JH. On the nature of the duality of the brain. In: Taylor J, ed. *Selected Writings of John Hughlings Jack-*

son. London, England: Hodder and Stoughton; 1982;2: 129–145.
20. Diamond M. Age, sex and environmental influences on anatomical asymmetry in rat forebrain. In: Geschwind N, Galaburda AM, eds. *Cerebral Dominance: The Biological Foundations.* Cambridge, Mass: Harvard University Press; 1994.
21. Brown JW. Rethinking the right hemisphere. In: Perecman E, ed. *Cognitive Processing in the Right Hemisphere.* New York, NY: Academic Press, Inc; 1983:41–53.
22. Gianotti G, Tiacci C. Patterns of drawing disability in right and left hemispheric patients. *Neuropsychologia.* 1970;8:379–384.
23. Warrington EK, James M, Kinsbourne M. Drawing disability in relation to laterality of cerebral lesion. *Brain.* 1966;89:53–82.
24. Levin HS. The acalculias. In: Heilman KM, Valenstein E, eds. *Clinical Neuropsychology.* New York, NY: Oxford University Press; 1979:128–140.
25. Butters N. Amnestic disorders. In: Heilman KM, Valenstein E, eds. *Clinical Neuropsychology.* New York, NY: Oxford University Press; 1979:439–474.
26. Geschwind N. The apraxias: Neural mechanisms of disorders of learned movements. *Am Sci.* 1975;63;188–195.
27. Ellis HD. The role of the right hemisphere in face perception. In: Young AW, ed. *Functions of the Right Cerebral Hemisphere.* New York, NY: Academic Press, Inc; 1983: 33–64.
28. Bogen JE. The other side of the brain. II: An appositional mind. *Bull Los Angeles Neurol Soc.* 1969;34:135–162.
29. Bradshaw JL, Nettleton NC. The nature of hemispheric specialization in man. *Behav Brain Sci.* 1981;4:51–91.
30. Bryden MP. *Laterality: Functional Asymmetry in the Intact Brain.* New York, NY: Academic Press, Inc; 1982.
31. Semmes J. Hemispheric specialization: A possible clue to mechanism. *Neuropsychologia.* 1968;6:11–26.

Chapter 2

Neurological Syndromes Associated with Right Hemisphere Damage

Jeffrey L. Cummings and Martha S. Burns

INTRODUCTION

Damage to the right hemisphere results in some of the most bizarre and complex syndromes observed in clinical medicine. Visual hallucinations, denial of illness, and disturbances of speech prosody are among the unusual symptoms exhibited by patients with injuries lateralized to the right side of the brain. This chapter presents the anatomical and biochemical differences between the two hemispheres and describes the clinical syndromes resulting from unilateral right hemisphere damage.

ANATOMICAL AND BIOCHEMICAL DIFFERENCES BETWEEN THE HEMISPHERES

The two hemispheres have been known to differ functionally since 1861 when Paul Broca noted that left-sided lesions produced aphasia whereas right hemisphere lesions did not (see Chapter 1). Despite this obvious functional difference, however, the two hemispheres were considered to be structurally identical until the seminal anatomical observations of Norman Geschwind and Walter Levitsky in 1968.[1] By systematically exposing the superior surface of the temporal lobe, they discovered that the planum temporale (the posterior area behind Heschl's gyrus) is larger on the left in 65% of brains and larger on the right in only 11%. Thus, the region of the brain crucially involved with language in the left hemisphere was consistently larger than in the contralateral hemisphere.

These original observations have been confirmed and expanded by other investigators. Gross anatomical asymmetries between the hemispheres include the configuration of the Sylvian fissures, the size and shape of the cerebral ventricles, the overall shape of the cerebral hemispheres, the volume of the anterior speech region, and the mode of crossing of the pyramidal tracts at their decussation in the medulla (Table 2–1).[2] The Sylvian fissure divides the temporal lobe from the overlying frontal and parietal lobes. On the left, the fissure continues smoothly posteriorly, whereas the right angulates superiorly in the posterior region. This anatomical divergence is visible at autopsy and can also be identified on angiograms demonstrating the course of the cerebral vessels that lie within the Sylvian fissures. The different positioning of the right and left Sylvian fissures creates a larger planum temporale on the left and a larger inferior parietal region on the right.[3,4]

Computed tomography and magnetic resonance imaging of the head reveal asymmetries in the cerebral ventricles. Between 60% and 70% of indi-

Table 2–1 Anatomical and Biochemical Differences Between the Left and Right Hemispheres

	Characteristic	Hemisphere Asymmetry
Gross Anatomy	Planum temporale	Larger on the left
	Anterior language area	Larger on the left
	Hemisphere shape	Longer and wider in left occipital lobe and right frontal lobe
	Sylvian fissures	Extend more posteriorly on the left and more superiorly on the right
	Lateral ventricles	Body and temporal horn wider on the left, occipital horn longer on the left
	Pyramidal tract	Larger left pyramidal tract crosses above the right in the medullary decussation
Histology (Cytoarchitectonics)	Planum temporale	Larger histologic area on the left
	Posterior thalamus	Larger on the left
	Auditory thalamus	Larger on the right
Biochemistry	Acetyltransferase	More concentrated in left temporal lobe
	Norepinephrine	More concentrated in left posterior nuclei and right somatosensory nuclei
	γ-Aminobutyric acid	Greater concentrations in left thalamus and caudate nucleus and right substantia nigra, superior colliculus, and nucleus accumbens

viduals have larger left-sided lateral ventricles. The width of the body and temporal horn is larger than the right, and the left occipital horn is longer.[5,6] Asymmetries also exist for the anterior speech regions (Broca's area) between the left and right hemispheres. Although the exterior portions of the regions are of equal size, when the intrasulcal surfaces are also included, a significant interhemispheric difference emerges, with the left side larger than the right.[7]

The two hemispheres are of different shapes. In a majority of brains, the left hemisphere has a longer and wider occipitoparietal area and the right hemisphere has a longer frontal lobe. These asymmetries are determined by measuring the indentations made on the internal surface of the skull by the underlying brain (as revealed by computed tomography) and they correlate well with the hemispheric asymmetries found at autopsy.[8-10]

The descending pyramidal tracts cross at the level of the medullary decussation. It is this decussation that underlies control of the right arm and leg by the right hemisphere. This decussation is asymmetrical, with the fibers crossing from left to right at a higher level in a majority of cases.[11]

The gross differences between the left and right hemispheres are visible in fetuses by 29 to 31 weeks' gestation and on endocasts of Neanderthal skulls that are 40,000 years old.[3,5,12-14] Similar, but less marked, differences occur in the brains of chimpanzees and orangutans.[15,16]

Histologic studies also reveal differences between the right and left hemispheres (see Table 2–1). Cytoarchitectonic investigations demonstrate that histologic boundaries correspond to the gross asymmetries of the temporal lobes described previously.[2] Such studies also reveal that the thalamic nuclei (lateral posterior) projecting to larger left hemisphere regions are of correspondingly greater size, and that those (medial geniculate) projecting to right-sided areas are increased in volume on the right.[17]

Biochemical asymmetries between the two hemispheres have received less attention and the results are less consistent (see Table 2–1). In humans, choline acetyltransferase concentrations are greater in the left temporal lobe than in the right.[18] The distribution of norepinephrine is more complex: its concentrations are greater in the posterior nuclei on the left and in the somatosensory nuclei on the right.[19] In the rat, concentrations of gamma-aminobutyric acid are higher in the left thalamus and caudate nucleus and the right substantia nigra, superior colliculus, and nucleus accumbens.[20]

Thus, while being of overall similar size and shape, the two hemispheres harbor a variety of anatomical and biochemical differences. Most of the asymmetries involve regions of the brain concerned with language mediation and show a bias toward increased size of the left temporal and inferior frontal regions. The posterior region, an area vitally concerned with visuospatial function, is larger on the right. In addition to the gross anatomical asymmetries, there are also interhemispheric differences in histologic structure and in the distribution of neurotransmitters. The asymmetries appear in the last trimester of gestation and were present in our Neanderthal ancestors.

CLINICAL SYNDROMES ASSOCIATED WITH RIGHT HEMISPHERE LESIONS

The neurobehavioral syndromes associated with lateralized right-sided lesions include attentional disorders, visuoperceptual deficits, visuomotor abnormalities, affective alterations, memory disturbances, and neuropsychiatric disorders (see Exhibit 2–1).

Attentional Disorders

Hemispatial Neglect

Hemispatial neglect refers to the failure of patients to distribute attention and to explore one side of space.[21] The symptoms that result are failure to detect, report, or orient to stimuli on one side of the body.[22] The neglected hemispace is contralateral to the lesion and occurs with parietal,

---

Exhibit 2–1 Classification of Clinical Syndromes Associated with Right Hemisphere Lesions

Attentional disturbances
- impaired distribution of attention in space
- impaired selective attention, especially for objects in space
- impaired vigilance

Visuoperceptual disturbances
- simultanagnosia
- achromatopsia
- environmental agnosia
- facial recognition deficits
- prosopagnosia

Visuomotor disturbances
- constructional disability
- dressing disturbances

Affective and emotional alterations
- anosognosia
- aprosody
- impaired affective auditory comprehension
- disturbance of emotional facial recognition
- altered emotional facial expression

Memory disturbances
- working memory disturbances
- decreased memory for nonverbal sequences
- recency and frequency judgment problems
- social/emotional memory problems
- nonverbal amnesia
- reduplicative paramnesia

Neuropsychiatric disorders
- visual hallucinations
- Capgras' syndrome
- secondary mania
- acute confusional states
- paranoid hallucinatory states

frontal, and subcortical lesions, although it is most profound with parietal lobe damage.[23,24] Hemispatial neglect may follow damage to left-sided as well as right-sided structures but is more severe and persistent with right-sided damage.

Unilateral neglect manifests itself in a variety of ways. The patient may fail to attend to somatosensory, auditory, or visual stimuli on one side. When the deficit is mild, the neglect is evident only when both sides are stimulated simultaneously; in more profound cases, all lateralized stimuli go undetected. The patient fails to orient to stimuli originating in the neglected hemispace and may ignore or turn away from examiners approaching from the neglected side. When asked to copy figures, the patient may see and reproduce only one half of the model, and when asked to cross lines distributed randomly on a page, the patient will cross only the lines in the nonneglected hemispace.[25] Hemialexia may result in reading only one half of words and sentences: "northwest" will be read as "west" and "baseball" will be read as "ball."[26] Hemiacalculia may occur when only one half of a series of numbers is included in the calculation process. The patient will also perceive only one half of the environment and may become lost from missing all turns in the neglected hemispace.[27]

Hemispatial neglect tends to be most profound in the initial phase of acute right-sided lesions. The neglect may resolve over time but is commonly still detectable many months later.[28] Hemispatial neglect is independent of the existence of a visual field defect: patients with neglect may have no field defect, and patients with visual field deficits may have no hemispatial neglect.[29]

Impaired Selective Attention and Vigilance

Selective attention refers to the ability to focus attention on a specific stimulus while inhibiting focus on competing or background stimuli. Attention can be directed toward a perceptual stimulus or a motor act. It is by nature fleeting and easily shifted to allow scanning the mental and external environment for relevant and interesting information while carrying out appropriate behavioral responses. Selective attentional circuits in the brain appear to involve the thalamus, which activates specific cortical regions while adjacent areas are suppressed, and the right dorsolateral prefrontal lobe, which appears important in selective attention to objects in space.[30,31]

Vigilance is a component of selective attention that permits a background readiness for relevant stimulus changes. Right hemisphere lesions impair selective attention by interfering with the activation of specific perceptual mechanisms. In addition, the ventromedial and dorsolateral prefrontal lobe component of right hemisphere attentional circuits become interrupted and affect working memory, vigilance, selective attention for objects and space, as well as some executive function aspects of attention such as planning and sequencing motor responses. These attentional disturbances become manifest as inattention to objects and spatial attributes of objects, impulsivity, distractibility, and disturbances in working memory.[31,32]

Visuoperceptual Disorders

Achromatopsia

Central achromatopsia refers to the loss of color vision produced by a brain lesion. It is limited to the hemifield contralateral to the lesion, and the necessary lesion is situated in the inferiomedial occipital region anterior to the visual cortex.[33] Infarction in the distribution of the posterior cerebral artery is the most common cause of central achromatopsia, but the syndrome has been produced by brain tumors and other focal lesions involving the ventromedial occipital cortex.[34,35]

Environmental Agnosia

Environmental agnosia is a unique syndrome manifested by a loss of environmental familiarity and an inability to become topographically oriented even in familiar surroundings.[36,37] Patients are able to see and accurately describe the environment, and their intellect and memory are unimpaired. Many develop verbal strategies to compensate for their recognition difficulties (e.g., "My bedroom is the third door on the left beyond the nurses' station.").

The origin of the recognition deficit is controversial, with some investigators viewing it as an amnesia and others championing the idea that it is an agnosia.[38,39] In many cases, however, memory is intact, and patients with memory disturbances do not exhibit the syndrome. The deficit appears to result from an inability to match intact perceptions with completely or partially preserved memory stores. This matching process is necessary to allow recognition and to impart a sense of familiarity to one's percepts. Thus, loss of environmental familiarity shares with other agnosias the essential feature of being a percept stripped of its meaning and is best classified as an environmental agnosia.

The lesion necessary to produce environmental agnosia is an inferiomedial temporo-occipital lesion in the right hemisphere. Although most patients have had right posterior cerebral artery infarctions, the syndrome has occurred with other etiologies.[40]

Facial Recognition Defects and Prosopagnosia

Defects in the recognition of famous faces, of matching two identical faces from a series of similar faces, and of choosing a previously seen face from among a group of faces are all more common with right hemisphere lesions than with left hemisphere lesions and more common with posterior damage than with anterior damage.[41–43] Tests with split-brain patients suggest that the right hemisphere is normally superior to the left in encoding complex stimuli (such as faces) that cannot be adequately differentiated with a verbal description, and that this skill is aborted by right hemisphere damage.[44]

Prosopagnosia is the failure to recognize familiar faces such as friends and members of one's own family. Recognition of familiar and discrimination of unfamiliar faces depend on independent central nervous system mechanisms, and lesions may produce defects in one ability without impairing the other.[45] Prosopagnosia has usually been attributed to bilateral lesions of the posterior hemispheres, and nearly all autopsied cases have had lesions of both hemispheres.[46,47] Prosopagnosia has occurred, however, in patients with computed tomographic evidence of unilateral right-sided lesions and in patients with unilateral surgical lesions, suggesting that appropriately placed lesions in the right hemisphere may be sufficient to disrupt the recognition of familiar as well as the discrimination of unfamiliar faces.[48,49]

Simultanagnosia

Simultanagnosia refers to the inability to perceive simultaneously the multiple details of a visual display. It is sometimes referred to as visual disorientation[21] and is one type of apperceptive object agnosia.[50] Patients with right hemisphere lesions often demonstrate this disturbance, which is manifest as inability to recognize objects as a whole. Instead of naming whole objects, the individual will describe visual features of the objects. The perceptual disturbance may underlie some of the other visuoperceptual problems discussed in this section, such as prosopagnosia.

Visuomotor Disorders

Constructional Disability

Constructional disability refers to the inability to draw spontaneously, copy model figures, reproduce geometric patterns with match sticks, or assemble blocks to imitate a model. There is a disturbance of assembling or articulating the parts that cannot be accounted for on the basis of visual, somatosensory, or motor deficits. Although often called constructional "apraxia," the disability does not meet the definition of apraxia as an inability to perform on command an act that can be performed spontaneously.[51]

Unilateral lesions of either the right or left hemisphere may give rise to constructional disability, and the deficits are more profound with posterior than with anterior lesions.[52–54] Qualitative differences between the drawings produced by patients with right hemisphere lesions have been observed. Right hemisphere damage results in a tendency to neglect the left half of models, to make errors in spatial relations, and to overscore existing lines and add extraneous material. Patients with left hemisphere injury produce simplified drawings.[55–57] While consistently present, the differences between the drawings produced by patients with right and left hemisphere damage are not sufficiently distinctive to allow differentiation of lateralized lesions solely on the basis of the constructional product.

Dressing Disturbances

There are two types of dressing disturbances: one in which the patient suffers from severe unilateral neglect and fails to dress one half of the body, and one in which body-garment disorientation makes it impossible for the patient to align body and clothes correctly. In the latter, the patient frequently turns the garment backward or inside-out, inverts right and left or top and bottom, and is able to conquer the logistics of dressing only with great difficulty. Body-garment disorientation has a virtually unique association with right parietal lobe damage.[58]

Affective and Emotional Alterations

The right hemisphere has often been regarded as the "emotional hemisphere," mediating human emotional life. This hypothesis is too broad and is being progressively refined to determine which components of emotion depend on right hemisphere integrity. Antonio Damasio[31] has studied the role of the right hemisphere in mediating emotion and has hypothesized, based on neuroimaging and lesion studies, that there is a specific social-emotional problem-solving circuit that includes the somatesthetic association areas of the right hemisphere; the amygdala (which is part of the limbic system), and the dorsolateral and ventromedial regions of the prefrontal cortex. The circuit processes information needed for learning and reasoning from social experience. The right somatesthetic cortex, at the same time, appears dominant for perception of emotional experience (i.e., mediating awareness of emotional experience processed by the limbic system). Damasio attributes many of the symptoms of right hemisphere dysfunction, including anosognosia and problems with social interaction, to damage in this circuitry. Other emotional functions mediated by the right hemisphere, which may or may not be damaged by damage to this circuit, include prosody of speech, affective auditory comprehension, recognition of emotional facial expression, comprehension of nonverbal gestural and paralinguistic cues, and emotional facial displays.

Anosognosia

Anosognosia refers to the denial of illness and frequently occurs to some degree in patients with hemispatial neglect.[59] The most common form occurs with right parietal lesions and involves denial of contralateral hemiparesis, hemisensory loss, or visual field defect. The neurobiological etiology of anosognosia is unknown, but Damasio[31] speculates that the right parietal lobe somatesthetic association cortex is dominant for body concept and awareness of emotional responses; impairment of these abilities may result in the anosognosia associated with right parietal lesions. The anosognosia varies from a simple underestimation of the degree of the deficit to a frank denial of any abnormality. In addition to denial of deficits, anosognosia also embraces a variety of unusual attitudes directed at the paretic limbs. Some patients minimize the deficits and joke about them (anosodiaphoria), some attribute ownership of the limbs to someone else (somatophrenia), some express hatred of the limb (misoplegia), and some exaggerate the strength of the limb (anosognosic overestimation).[60] A related phenomenon is the false belief that an additional limb has appeared on the paralyzed side.[61]

Anosognosia may constitute a considerable barrier to rehabilitation since the patient who is unaware of any deficit is unlikely to be successfully engaged in therapy.

Aprosody

Prosody refers to the affective coloring, melody, and cadence of speech. These nonverbal aspects of communication impart linguistic (sometimes called intrinsic) information and emotional content to propositional speech. Prosody thus allows communication of such information as signaling the end of a statement or turn, and the type of information being shared (e.g., question or statement). It also allows communication of the intent, mood, and interest level of the speaker. Normal linguistic prosody depends on both left and right hemispheric integrity, but right-sided lesions may impair emotional prosody without altering the propositional component of verbal output. Motor prosody is impaired by anteriorly placed lesions in the right hemisphere.[62–65]

Impaired Affective Auditory Comprehension

Variously called *affective auditory agnosia*[66] and *receptive aprosodia*,[65,67] comprehension of the affective or prosodic elements of speech is also dependent on the right hemisphere. Patients with right parietal lesions fail to comprehend the prosodic speech elements but have no impairment of propositional language comprehension. Such patients also have difficulty repeating the affective intonation of sample sentences provided by the examiner.[68,69]

Disturbances of Emotional Facial Recognition

As noted previously, the right hemisphere is superior to the left on tasks of facial recognition and facial discrimination. It has been difficult to dissociate recognition of faces from recognition of facial expressions, but evidence is consistent in demonstrating that the patient with right hemisphere damage is disadvantaged in the recognition and interpretation of emotional expressions.[70]

Altered Emotional Facial Expression

Human emotions are expressed more intensely on the left side than on the right side of the face, suggesting an asymmetrical control of facial expression with a right-sided predominance.[31,71] Lateralized right-sided lesions are thus more likely than left-sided lesions to impair facial displays of emotional expression.

Memory Disorders

Disturbances of Working Memory

The right dorsolateral prefrontal lobe appears to permit holding of visually perceived information briefly so that cognitive operations can be performed on the percept. This is known as *working memory*. Working memory for objects in space permits holding of spatial attributes of objects for executive function operations.[72,73] As noted previously, right hemisphere lesions interrupt the attentional and social-emotional problem-solving circuits that connect the dorsolateral frontal lobes and the right somatesthetic association cortex. This circuitry disruption is presumed to be the cause of problems with working memory exhibited by patients with right hemisphere lesions.[30–32] These patients often have particular difficulty holding visual information in mind while performing a cognitive operation on the information. Working memory is thought to be important in solving problems of everyday life, especially making and holding visual plans of action to tackle logistically difficult situations, like planning how one could carry two large suitcases onto a plane while handing the flight attendant the ticket.[30] This impairment might also explain why patients with right hemisphere lesions show impulsivity on motor responses and evidence difficulties with motor planning.

Problems with Recency and Frequency Judgments

In addition to their role in executive function and working memory, the dorsolateral prefrontal lobes are important to memory for how recently an event has occurred and how frequently it occurs (recency and frequency judgments).[73] Again, perhaps because of the interruption of the right hemisphere circuitry that connects the amygdala with the dorsolateral prefrontal lobes and the right somatesthetic cortex, persons with right hemisphere damage often show problems with memory for recency and frequency. They forget when they last participated in an action or event (e.g., when a medication was last taken or when a treatment was last administered) and they forget how often or how long it occurred (e.g., how frequently they received one therapy or another).

Problems with Retention of Visual Sequences

The right thalamus is important to retention of the sequences of visual events.[31] Those with right hemisphere brain damage, presumably because of the interruption of thalamic circuitry on the right, often have problems retaining sequences that require visualization (such as daily schedules or the sequence of steps required to perform visually planned operations such as changing a light bulb).

Nonverbal Amnesia

Right hemisphere lesions preferentially affect the recall of nonverbal visual material. Right temporal lobectomy results in impairment of retention of complex visual patterns and faces.[74] Right thalamic lesions also disrupt nonverbal memory in contrast to the impairment of verbal memory produced by left-sided temporal lobe and thalamic lesions.[75,76]

Reduplicative Paramnesia

Reduplicative paramnesia or environmental reduplication is a disorder of spatial orientation in which the patient insists that a current unfamiliar environment (e.g., the hospital) is located closer to a place that is more important and familiar (e.g., home).[77-79] The complex confabulation syndrome appears to depend on a combination of impaired spatial perception, poor visual memory, and inability to recognize the dissonance in responses. These patients have most commonly had a combination of right parietal and bilateral frontal injuries or right parietal damage and an acute confusional state.

Neuropsychiatric Disorders

Visual Hallucinations

Visual hallucinations can be operationally defined as a symptom in which the patient claims to see or behaves as if he sees something that the observer cannot see.[80] Visual hallucinations associated with lesions within the hemisphere may be ictal in origin, occurring as part of a focal seizure, or they may be release hallucinations associated with visual field defects. Release hallucinations occur with right-sided lesions and are frequent with lesions involving the posterior aspect of the hemisphere.[81,82] The hallucinatory visions tend to begin soon after an acute cerebral insult, occur in the region of a visual field defect, persist for several hours at a time, consist of formed images of animals or persons, and gradually abate after several months. The patient usually appreciates the hallucinatory nature of the images.

Pallinopsia is a special variant of release hallucination in which the major feature is the abnormal persistence or recurrence of visual images after the exciting stimulus has been removed.[83] After looking away from the face or object, the original image persists for up to several minutes and may spontaneously recur several hours later. Pallinopsia has the same association with lesions of the right posterior hemisphere that is noted with typical release hallucinations.[84,85]

Capgras' Syndrome

Capgras' syndrome is the delusional belief that individuals close to one have been replaced by identical-appearing impostors. The patient can detect no physical changes that distinguish the impostor, but the patient is convinced that an impersonation is occurring. Capgras' syndrome is often part of a complex persecutory delusion in which the patient believes that the impostor is perpetrating the masquerade in order to obtain money or property illegally. Many patients with Capgras' syndrome have right hemisphere damage, and the syndrome has been observed in patients with post-traumatic encephalopathy, epilepsy, cerebrovascular disease, and a variety of other neurological disorders.[86–88]

Secondary Mania

Secondary mania refers to an elated and/or irritable mood lasting at least 1 week and combined with at least two of the following: hyperactivity, pressured speech, flight of ideas, grandiosity, diminished sleep, distractibility, and lack of judgment.[89] Secondary mania may be induced by specific drugs (e.g., levodopa, corticosteroids), by metabolic disturbances (e.g., hemodialysis), and by focal brain insults. Nearly all focal central nervous system lesions producing mania have been located in the right cerebral hemisphere, and most of the lesions have been in deep midline regions adjacent to the third ventricle.[90] The acute onset of mania in a patient over the age of 40 with no history of an affective disorder should raise consideration of secondary mania. Patients with right hemisphere lesions may be at increased risk for the development of mania.

Acute Confusional States

Confusional states are usually the result of an encephalopathy produced by a toxic or metabolic disturbance of brain function. In a few cases, however, confusional states have resulted from focal brain insults. The two focal syndromes associated with confusion are bilateral temporo-occipital lesions and right middle cerebral artery infarctions.[91,92] The latter produce profound deficits in attention without significantly depressing arousal. The confusional state resolves in 1 to 3 weeks and is attributable to interruption of the dominant attentional functions of the right hemisphere.

Paranoid Hallucinatory States

Right hemisphere lesions may also give rise to paranoid hallucinatory states. The patients suffer from persecutory delusions and ideas of reference and have auditory and visual hallucinations. The psychosis has schizophrenia-like features and closely resembles idiopathic psychosis. In most cases, the lesions associated with paranoid hallucinatory states have involved the right temporoparietal region and have been produced by vascular occlusions.[93,94]

COMMENT

The functions of the right cerebral hemisphere are complex and diverse and can be regarded as *nondominant* or *minor* only with regard to the linguistic abilities of the left hemisphere. For many skills, the right hemisphere has superior abilities. No single characteristic appears to summarize adequately the function of the right hemisphere or account for the variety of deficits that follow right hemisphere insults. Spatial and social-affective functions dominate the activities of the right hemisphere: in the spatial realm the right hemisphere mediates visuoperceptual function, visuomotor activities, and visuospatial memory; in the realm of social-affective function its integrity is necessary for the production and perception of emotional facial expression and emotional sound inflection. Flor-Henry[95] has suggested that these spatial and affective functions may share a common evolutionary history, with the visuospatial abilities concerned with territorial surveillance and the affective displays involved in territorial protection. These functions may have originally occupied both hemispheres and may have become lateralized to the right by the asymmetrical acquisition of language abilities by the left hemisphere.

Whatever the evolutionary background of the right hemisphere function, damage to this cerebral member gives rise to complex neurobehavioral syndromes that may include disturbances of perception, constructions, dressing, and memory, as well as neuropsychiatric syndromes such as hallucinations, Capgras' syndrome, and mania.

REFERENCES

1. Geschwind N, Levitsky W. Human brain: Left-right asymmetries in temporal speech region. *Science*. 1968; 161:186–187.

2. Galaburda AM, LeMay M, Kemper TL, et al. Right-left asymmetries in the brain. *Science*. 1978;199:852–856.

3. LeMay M, Culebras A. Human brain—morphologic differences in the hemispheres demonstrable by carotid arteriography. *N Engl J Med.* 1972;287:168–170.
4. Rubens AB, Mahowald MW, Hutton JT. Asymmetry of the lateral (sylvian) fissures in man. *Neurology.* 1976;26:620–624.
5. LeMay M. Morphological cerebral asymmetries of modern man, fossil man, and non-human primate. *Ann NY Acad Sci.* 1976;280:349–366.
6. Greenberg JO, ed. *Neuroimaging.* New York, NY: McGraw-Hill Publishing Co; 1995.
7. Falzi G, Perrone P, Vignolo LA. Right-left asymmetry in anterior speech regions. *Arch Neurol.* 1982;39:239–240.
8. LeMay M. Asymmetries of the skull and handedness. *J Neurol Sci.* 1977;32:243–253.
9. Pieniadz JM, Naeser MA. Computed tomographic scan cerebral asymmetries and morphologic brain asymmetries. *Arch Neurol.* 1984;41:403–409.
10. Weinberger DR, Luchins DJ, Morisha J, Wyatt RJ. Asymmetrical volumes of the right and left frontal and occipital regions of the human brain. *Ann Neurol.* 1982;11:97–100.
11. Kertesz A, Geschwind N. Patterns of pyramidal decussation and their relationship to handedness. *Arch Neurol.* 1971;24:326–332.
12. Chi Je G, Dooling EC, Gilles FH. Left-right asymmetries of the temporal speech areas of the human fetus. *Arch Neurol.* 1979;34:346–348.
13. Wada JA, Clarke R, Hamm A. Cerebral hemispheric asymmetry in humans. *Arch Neurol.* 1975;32:239–246.
14. Witelson SF, Pallie W. Left hemisphere specialization for language in the newborn. *Brain.* 1973;96:641–646.
15. LeMay M, Geschwind N. Hemispheric differences in the brains of great apes. *Brain Behav Evol.* 1975;11:48–52.
16. Yeni-Komshian GH, Benson DA. Anatomical study of cerebral asymmetry in the temporal lobe of humans, chimpanzees and rhesus monkeys. *Science.* 1976;192:387–389.
17. Eidelberg D, Galaburda AM. Symmetry and asymmetry in the human posterior thalamus. *Arch Neurol.* 1982;39:325–332.
18. Amaducci L, Sorbi S, Albanese A, et al. Choline acetyltransferase (CHAT) activity differs in right and left human temporal lobes. *Neurology.* 1981;31:799–805.
19. Oke A, Keller R, Mefford I, et al. Lateralization of norepinephrine in human thalamus. *Science.* 1978;200:1411–1413.
20. Starr MS, Kilpatrick IC. Bilateral asymmetry in brain GABA function? *Neurosci Lett.* 1981;25:167–172.
21. Mesulam MM. Attention, confusional states and neglect. In: Mesulam MM, ed. *Principles of Behavioral Neurology.* Philadelphia, Pa: FA Davis Co; 1985:125–168.
22. Heilman KM. Neglect and related disorders. In: Heilman KM, Valenstein E, eds. *Clinical Neuropsychology.* New York, NY: Oxford University Press; 1979:268–307.
23. Mesulam MM. A cortical network for directed attention and unilateral neglect. *Ann Neurol.* 1981;10:309–325.
24. Watson RT, Heilman KM. Thalamic neglect. *Neurology.* 1979;29:690–694.
25. Albert ML. A simple test of visual neglect. *Neurology.* 1973;23:658–664.
26. Henderson VW, Alexander MP, Naeser MA. Right thalamic injury, impaired visuospatial perception, and alexia. *Neurology.* 1982;32:235–240.
27. Brain WR. Visual disorientation with special reference to lesions of the right cerebral hemisphere. *Brain.* 1941;64:244–272.
28. Colombo A, DeRenzi E, Gentilini M. The time course of visual hemi-inattention. *Arch Psychiatr Nervenkr.* 1982;231:539–546.
29. Willanger R, Danielsen UT, Ankerhus J. Visual neglect in right-sided apoplectic lesions. *Acta Neurol Scand.* 1981;64:327–336.
30. LaBerge D. *Attentional Processing.* Cambridge, Mass: Harvard University Press; 1995.
31. Damasio A. *Descartes' Error: Emotion, Reason and the Human Brain.* New York, NY: Grosset, Putnam; 1994.
32. Tompkins CA, Bloise C, Timko ML, Baumgaertner A. Working memory and inference revision in brain-damaged and normally aging adults. *J Speech and Hearing Research.* 1994;37:896–913.
33. Damasio A, Yamada T, Damasio H, et al. Central achromatopsia: Behavioral, anatomic, and physiologic aspects. *Neurology.* 1980;30:1064–1071.
34. Green GJ, Lessell S. Acquired cerebral dyschromatopsia. *Arch Ophthalmol.* 1977;95:121–128.
35. Meadows JC. Disturbed perceptions of colours associated with localized cerebral lesions. *Brain.* 1974;97:615–632.
36. McFie J, Piercy MF, Zangwill OL. Visual-spatial agnosia associated with lesions of the right cerebral hemisphere. *Brain.* 1950;73:167–190.
37. Paterson A, Zangwill OL. A case of topographical disorientation associated with a unilateral cerebral lesion. *Brain.* 1945;68:188–212.
38. Hecaen H, Tzortzis C, Rondot P. Loss of topographic memory with learning deficits. *Cortex.* 1980;16:525–542.
39. Whiteley AM, Warrington EK. Selective impairment of topographical memory: A single case study. *J Neurol Neurosurg Psychiatry.* 1978;41:575–578.
40. Cogan D. Visuospatial dysgnosia. *Am J Ophthalmol.* 1979;88:361–368.
41. DeRenzi E, Scotti G, Spinnler H. Perceptual and associative disorders in visual recognition. *Neurology.* 1969;19:634–642.

42. Warrington EK, James M. An experimental investigation of facial recognition in patients with unilateral cerebral lesions. *Cortex.* 1967;3:317–326.
43. Van Lancker DR, Canter GJ. Impairment of voice and face recognition in patients with hemispheric damage. *Brain Cognit.* 1982;1:185–195.
44. Gazzaniga MS, Smylie CS. Facial recognition and brain asymmetries: Clues to underlying mechanisms. *Ann Neurol.* 1983;13:536–540.
45. Malone DR, Morris HH, Kay MC, et al. Prosopagnosia: A double dissociation between the recognition of familiar and unfamiliar faces. *J Neurol Neurosurg Psychiatry.* 1982;45:820–822.
46. Cohn R, Neumann MA, Wood DH. Prosopagnosia: A clinicopathological study. *Ann Neurol.* 1977;1:177–182.
47. Meadows JC. The anatomical basis of prosopagnosia. *J Neurol Neurosurg Psychiatry.* 1974;37:489–501.
48. Hecaen H, Angelergues R. Agnosia for faces (prosopagnosia). *Arch Neurol.* 1962;7:92–100.
49. Whiteley AM, Warrington EK. Prosopagnosia: A clinical, psychological, and anatomical study of three patients. *J Neurol Neurosurg Psychiatry.* 1977;40:395–403.
50. McCarthy RA, Warrington EK. *Cognitive Neuropsychology.* New York, NY: Academic Press, Inc; 1990.
51. Geschwind N. The apraxias: Neural mechanisms of disorders of learned movement. *Am Sci.* 1975;63:188–195.
52. Arena R, Gianotti G. Constructional apraxia and visuoperceptive disabilities in relation to laterality of cerebral lesions. *Cortex.* 1978;14:463–473.
53. Benson DF, Barton MI. Disturbances in constructional ability. *Cortex.* 1970;6:19–46.
54. Piercy M, Hecaen H, DeAjuriaguerra J. Constructional apraxia associated with unilateral cerebral lesions—left- and right-sided cases compared. *Brain.* 1960;83:225–242.
55. Arrigoni G, DeRenzi E. Constructional apraxia and hemispheric locus of lesion. *Cortex.* 1964;1:170–197.
56. Gianotti G, Tiacci C. Patterns of drawing disability in right and left hemispheric patients. *Neuropsychologia.* 1970;8:379–384.
57. Warrington EK, James M, Kinsbourne M. Drawing disability in relation to laterality of cerebral lesion. *Brain.* 1966;89:53–82.
58. Hemphill RE, Klein R. Contribution to the dressing disability as a focal sign and to the imperception phenomena. *J Ment Sci.* 1948;94:611–622.
59. Weinstein EA, Kahn RL. The syndrome of anosognosia. *Arch Neurol Psychiatry.* 1950;64:772–791.
60. Cutting J. Study of anosognosia. *J Neurol Neurosurg Psychiatry.* 1978;41:548–555.
61. Weinstein EA, Kahn RL, Malitz S, et al. Delusional reduplication of parts of the body. *Brain.* 1954;77:45–56.
62. Ross ED. The aprosodias. *Arch Neurol.* 1981;38:561–569.
63. Ross ED, Mesulam MM. Dominant language functions of the right hemisphere? *Arch Neurol.* 1979;36:144–148.
64. Weintraub S, Mesulam MM, Kramer L. Disturbances in prosody. *Arch Neurol.* 1981;38:742–744.
65. Ross E. Neurology of affect. Presented at Northwestern University Medical School Conference on Neurology and Cognition; December 15, 1994; Chicago, Ill.
66. Heilman KM, Bowers D, Speedie L, Coslett HB. The comprehension of emotional and nonemotional prosody. *Neurology.* 1984;34:917–921.
67. Ross E. Modulation of affect and nonverbal communication by the right hemisphere. In: Mesulam MM, ed. *Principles of Behavioral Neurology.* Philadelphia, Pa: FA Davis Co; 1985:239–257.
68. Heilman KM, Scholes R, Watson RT. Auditory affective agnosia. *J Neurol Neurosurg Psychiatry.* 1975;38:69–72.
69. Tucker DM, Watson RT, Heilman KM. Discrimination and evocation of affectively intoned speech in patients with right parietal disease. *Neurology.* 1977;27:947–950.
70. Dekosky ST, Heilman KM, Bowers D, et al. Recognition and discrimination of emotional faces and pictures. *Brain Lang.* 1980;9:206–214.
71. Sackheim HA, Gur RC, Saucy MC. Emotions are expressed more intensely on the left side of the face. *Science.* 1978;202:434–436.
72. Baddeley AD. *Working Memory.* Oxford, England: Oxford University Press; 1986.
73. Tranel D, Damasio AR. Neurobiological foundations of human memory. In: Baddeley AD, Wilson BA, Watts FN, eds. *Handbook of Memory Disorders.* New York, NY: John Wiley & Sons, Inc; 1995.
74. Milner B. Visual recognition and recall after right temporal lobe excision in man. *Neuropsychologia.* 1968;6:191–209.
75. Milner B. Psychological defects produced by temporal lobe excision. *Res Publ Assocn Res Nerv Ment Dis.* 1958;36:244–257.
76. Speedie LJ, Heilman KM. Anterograde memory deficits for visuospatial material after infarction of the right thalamus. *Arch Neurol.* 1983;40:183–186.
77. Benson DF, Gardner H, Meadows JC. Reduplicative paramnesia. *Neurology.* 1976;26:147–151.
78. Fisher CM. Disorientation for place. *Arch Neurol.* 1982;39:33–36.
79. Ruff RL, Volpe BT. Environmental reduplication associated with right frontal and parietal lobe injury. *J Neurol Neurosurg Psychiatry.* 1981;44:382–386.
80. Lessell S. Higher disorders of visual function: Positive phenomena. In: Glaser JS, Smith JL, eds. *Neuro-ophthalmology.* St. Louis, Mo: CV Mosby Co; 1975;8:27–44.

81. Brust JCM, Behrens MM. "Release hallucinations" as the major symptom of posterior cerebral artery occlusion: A report of 2 cases. *Ann Neurol.* 1977;2:432–436.

82. Lance JW. Simple formed hallucinations confined to the area of a specific visual field defect. *Brain.* 1976;99:719–734.

83. Bender MB, Feldman M, Sobin AJ. Palinopsia. *Brain.* 1968;91:321–338.

84. Cummings JL, Syndulko K, Goldberg Z, et al. Palinopsia reconsidered. *Neurology.* 1980;32:444–447.

85. Michel EM, Troost BT. Palinopsia: Cerebral localization with computed tomography. *Neurology.* 1980;30:887–889.

86. Alexander MP, Stuss DT, Benson DF. Capgras' syndrome: A reduplicative phenomenon. *Neurology.* 1979;29:334–339.

87. Cummings JL. Organic delusions: Phenomenology, anatomic correlations, and review. *Br J Psychiatry.* 1985;146:184–197.

88. Hayman MA, Abrams R. Capgras' syndrome and cerebral dysfunction. *Br J Psychiatry.* 1977;130:68–71.

89. Krauthammer C, Klerman GL. Secondary mania. *Arch Gen Psychiatry.* 1978;35:1333–1339.

90. Cummings JL, Mendez MF. Secondary mania with focal cerebrovascular lesions. *Am J Psychiatry.* 1984;141:1084–1087.

91. Medina JL, Chokroverty S, Rubino FA. Syndrome of agitated delirium and visual impairment: A manifestation of medial temporo-occipital infarction. *J Neurol Neurosurg Psychiatry.* 1977;40:861–864.

92. Mesulam MM, Waxman SG, Geschwind N, Sabin TD. Acute confusional states with right middle cerebral artery infarctions. *J Neurol Neurosurg Psychiatry.* 1976;39:84–89.

93. Levine DN, Finkelstein S. Delayed psychosis after right temporoparietal stroke or trauma: Relation to epilepsy. *Neurology.* 1982;32:267–273.

94. Peroutka SJ, Sohmer BH, Kumar AJ, et al. Hallucinations and delusions following a right temporo-parieto-occipital infarction. *Johns Hopkins Med J.* 1982;151:181–185.

95. Flor-Henry P. *Cerebral Basis of Psychopathology.* Boston, Mass: John Wright-PSG, Inc; 1983.

Chapter 3

A Conceptual Framework for the Evaluation and Treatment of Communication Problems Associated with Right Hemisphere Damage

Leora Reiff Cherney and Anita S. Halper

INTRODUCTION

Historically, it was thought that damage only to the left hemisphere, and not the right hemisphere, had an impact on communication skills.[1,2] However, recent evidence suggests that the right hemisphere makes an important contribution to language processing, and it is acknowledged widely that right hemisphere damage also results in impairments in communication.[3-7] In contrast to aphasia, communication problems associated with right hemisphere damage are not symbolic in nature, but rather a cluster of cognitive deficits that reduce the patient's effective and efficient communication skills.

Exhibit 3-1 illustrates the communicative interaction of three patients with right hemisphere damage. All of these verbal exchanges have two things in common. First, the basic linguistic elements—phonology, syntax, and lexical choices—are intact. Second, the responses do not adequately answer the questions asked. There are also some striking differences among the responses, with each utterance failing to communicate for different reasons. According to Burns,[3] J.K. interprets the clinician's question literally and attempts to answer how he was transported to his present location. However, he seems to have confused cities and train stations along the way. R.H. appears to have interpreted the intent of the question appropriately, but in trying to answer he becomes tangential about details of the evening and is unable to tie his story together or get back to the main topic. H.P. also seems to interpret the intent of the question but expresses a lack of understanding about why she is in the hospital and a misperception of her mode of transport.

The goal of this chapter is to review the current literature relevant to communication and cognition, in an attempt to provide an explanation for the breakdown in the effectiveness of communication illustrated in Exhibit 3-1. The ability to communicate effectively and efficiently is dependent on the integrity of both linguistic and cognitive processes.[8] The linguistic processes include phonology, morphology, syntax, semantics, and pragmatics. The cognitive processes include attention, perception, memory, organization, reasoning, and problem solving. Right hemisphere communication impairments are believed to result from deficits in any of these processes. Such cognitively based disorders of communication have been

Exhibit 3–1 Examples of Communicative Interactions

EXCHANGE 1

Clinician: Can you tell me how you got here?

J.K.: You won't believe it, but I took Amtrak from Las Vegas or rather from Kingston, Arizona, to Grand, Grand Union Station here in Vegas in Chicago.

EXCHANGE 2

Clinician: Could you tell me what happened to you when you came to the hospital?

R.H.: Well, I hear it more from others than I recollect it. Um, but two days beforehand we were out at the club. I was enjoying myself, maybe too much but I was enjoying myself. And suddenly I . . . my words began to slur and (my thoughts always slur but my words don't) and some man, Bill Williams, Dr. Bill Williams, he's on the staff isn't he? He sent word to my waitress that he would go down in the locker room and I oughta come down and have him check him out. So you can see what improvement there's been.

EXCHANGE 3

Clinician: Why did you have to come to the hospital?

H.P.: Well, I don't know. They say I fell and like that . . . so they didn't know what to do so the yard man, he asked the lady across the street what he should do, and she said well call the ambulance, but they wouldn't send no ambulance so they sent this . . . like a haywagon picked me up and brought me here.

referred to as *cognitive-communicative impairments*.[8]

This chapter presents a conceptual framework for the clinical management of cognitive-communicative impairments associated with right hemisphere damage. This framework has grown out of clinical experience with patients with right hemisphere damage. It is intended to be used as a clinical guide for selecting appropriate evaluation and treatment materials. It is not meant to be a theoretical model of brain organization and function. Figure 3–1 is a schematic representation of the interrelationships among different cognitive processes that may be affected by right hemisphere damage. First, each of the processes will be defined, and then the interrelationships between these processes and their impact on communication will be discussed.

The premise of this framework is that these processes underlie the performance of any functional behavior including communication. When communication breaks down in a specific task, the underlying reason for the problem needs to be analyzed. The clinician has several choices available for treatment, depending on the results of the evaluation. One choice may be to work on the presumed underlying cognitive process. A second option may be to work on the symptom or the resultant impaired functional behavior while simultaneously providing the patient with compensatory strategies to overcome the impaired underlying cognitive process. A third choice for clinicians is to adopt both of these options.

For example, a patient may have reading problems due to left neglect, or problems in visual perception, attention, and/or memory. If the underlying cause of the reading problem is difficulty sustaining attention, the clinician may choose to work on vigilance tasks that do not involve the actual task of reading. Or the clinician may provide the patient with cues to increase attentional skills while the patient is actually reading. If the underlying cause of the reading problem is left neglect, the clinician may work on reading while using compensatory strategies such as a red line on the left side of the page. Or the clinician may choose to work on left neglect in nonverbal perceptual tasks. Regardless of the option chosen for treat-

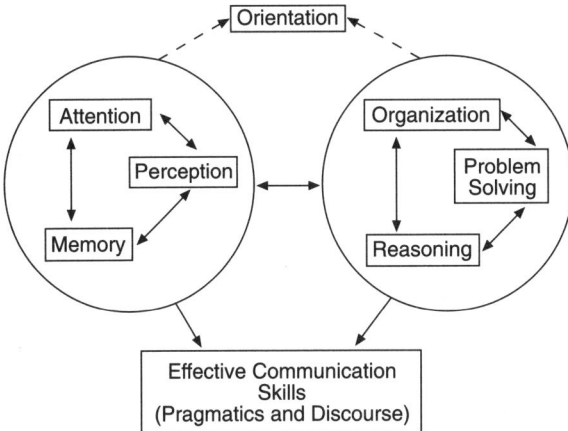

Figure 3–1 Schematic representation of interrelationships among cognitive processes

ment, the clinician needs to keep in mind the underlying reasons for the breakdown in communication.

COGNITIVE PROCESSES

Attention

Attention is a complex process that includes several components. Sohlberg and Mateer[9,10] delineate five levels of attention: focused, sustained, selective, alternating, and divided attention. Focused attention is the ability to direct attention to specific sensory stimuli. Sustained attention involves actively maintaining attention to the stimuli over a period of time. Selective attention is the ability to focus attention on target stimuli while ignoring irrelevant stimuli. Alternating attention is the ability to shift from one task to another task that requires different mental processes. Divided attention is the ability to focus and sustain attention on more than one task simultaneously.

Each individual has a finite attentional capacity and, therefore, the attentional resources need to be carefully controlled and allocated to effectively perform a task.[7] In patients with right hemisphere damage, attentional capacity may be reduced. This may result in decreased performance on complex tasks and difficulty focusing and sustaining attention to more than one task simultaneously (divided attention).

The most clinically significant disorder of attention that occurs when the right hemisphere is damaged is left-side neglect. The patient is not aware of and does not respond to stimuli in the left hemispace. Neglect is most common in the visual modality, but may occur in the auditory, olfactory, or tactile modality.[11] Neglect may appear more severe in tasks where the demands for selective attention are greater.[12]

Mesulam[11] describes why hemispatial neglect occurs more frequently following right hemisphere damage as compared to left hemisphere damage. He indicates that the intact left hemisphere is responsible for exploring and maintaining the awareness of the right side of space. On the other hand, the right hemisphere is responsible for exploring and maintaining awareness of both the left and right sides of space. When a lesion occurs in the left hemisphere, the intact right hemisphere is able to maintain directed attention to both sides of space. When a lesion occurs in the right hemisphere, the intact left hemisphere is able to maintain attention to the right side of space only, resulting in a left-side neglect.

Memory

Memory, like attention, is a complex process. Memory deficits are often a manifestation of brain damage and not the result of damage to a particular area of the brain. Therefore, any of the operations of memory discussed below may be impaired. In addition, patients with right hemisphere damage may show difficulty with nonverbal or spatial memory.[7]

The Operations of Memory

There are three operations of memory: encoding, storage, and retrieval.[13]

Encoding or memorizing is the set of processes by which the representation of an event is formed and constructed.[14] The memorizing process consists of two stages, a holding stage and an acquiring stage. The holding stage operates when the attention span is exceeded. If the holding stage is absent, the information is not processed or each new piece of information deletes the previous piece.

The acquiring stage consists of several steps.[14] First, information is analyzed superficially or deeply. Superficial analysis focuses on the sensory attributes such as how the target information sounds or looks. Deep analysis targets the semantic or conceptual characteristics. Subjects recall items that are deeply encoded better than items that are superficially encoded.[15] For example, subjects recall words better when they are asked questions about their meaning (Is it a piece of furniture?) rather than questions about the sound of the word (Does it rhyme with hair?).

Second, the quantity of information is reduced and organized. This is achieved by grouping and categorizing. Third, the information is associated with the context in which it occurred. Contextual cues related to the environment and the time of the event are used to facilitate this association. The acquiring process depends on the holding process. If the holding process is inadequate, then the acquiring process will be incomplete.

Storage is the process of transferring a transient memory into permanent storage. Two mechanisms, consolidation and reconstruction, are important for storage.[11] Consolidation is the integration of new information into the existing permanent memory store. Reconstruction is the reorganization and reassembling of memory traces within the permanent memory store as new memories are added.

During retrieval of information, memory traces are activated in the permanent store so they are available for use. Once they are activated, they must be chosen according to the situation. Retrieval can be explicit or implicit. When it is explicit, retrieval is conscious and voluntary. When it is implicit, retrieval is automatic without conscious awareness. Cues for partial bits of information can elicit retrieval of information without the individual being aware that the information was previously presented. This is referred to as *priming effects*.

Aspects of Memory

Clinically, the terms *short-* and *long-term memory* are often used. Short-term memory is the temporary storage system that holds information for a few seconds or minutes for either retrieval or transfer to the more permanent, long-term memory store. Long-term memory permanently stores knowledge and experience over various time periods ranging from minutes to years. This simple, dual model has both theoretical problems and clinical limitations. There are problems distinguishing between long- and short-term memory, such as length of time the memory trace remains in short-term memory. This model has not held well in experimental paradigms.[10]

A more dynamic concept that is related to short-term memory is that of *working memory*. It was initially proposed by Baddeley and Hitch[16] and incorporates both the holding and acquiring stages (i.e., capacity of holding information temporarily while performing mental operations). Rather than a unitary system, working memory is conceived of as a collection of work areas where information is temporarily processed simultaneously. Each cognitive processing system has its own working memory capacity that is integrated by a central executive system.[16] In the patient with right hemisphere damage, it has been proposed that working memory limitations may adversely affect performance on a variety of tasks.[17]

Long-term memory has been divided into several categories including semantic and episodic memory and procedural and declarative memory. Semantic memory (memory for knowledge including word meanings) is acquired independent of the situational context. For example, most people know that Washington, DC, is the capital of the United States, but most cannot recall when the information was acquired. Episodic memory is dependent on specific situations and events and allows one to remember past experiences. For example, remembering the people attending a birthday party and the gifts received is considered episodic memory.

Declarative memory requires conscious awareness. The individual must be able to explain specifically the event or task. Declarative memory seems to be similar to explicit memory. Procedural memory is the ability to perform the sequences of a task automatically, such as driving a car or operating a videocassette recorder. It is one aspect of implicit memory.

Another aspect of memory is retrospective memory, which is memory for events and information from the past. This contrasts with prospective memory, which is the ability to remember to do something at a future time. Therefore, prospective memory is essential for functioning in the environment on a day-to-day basis.

Perception

Perception is an active process that structures the environment by integrating sensory stimuli into meaningful units.[18] In patients with right hemisphere damage, both visual and auditory perceptual problems have been identified. Visual perceptual problems include such deficits as impaired face recognition, impaired figure-ground discrimination, impaired color recognition, and impaired scanning. Since the visual system is complex and widely distributed in the brain,[10] some problems such as color and shape recognition may occur only after bilateral hemisphere damage.[19] Auditory perceptual deficits include such problems as impaired perception of music and impaired perception of prosody.

Perceptual problems can lead to confusion and disorientation. According to Myers and Mackisack,[6] the patient with right hemisphere damage is able to "see" the elements, but has difficulty integrating them and evaluating them within the context. For example, one of our patients with right hemisphere stroke said: "I can see your eyelashes perfectly and your eyes and your teeth, but what good are those things without a body behind them."

Organization, Reasoning, and Problem Solving

Organization is the ability to sort, categorize, sequence, and prioritize information. The ability to determine likenesses and differences is required to organize information. Organization is fundamental to reasoning, problem solving, and judgment.[10]

Reasoning is the ability to think abstractly and draw inferences and conclusions based on known or supposed information. Patients with right hemisphere damage may have difficulty comprehending the meaning of abstract language such as jokes,[20,21] proverbs,[22] and indirect requests.[23–25]

Individuals reason in several ways. Inductive reasoning involves drawing conclusions from partial or indirect information. Deductive reasoning involves logically determining specific facts from a general premise or principle. In deductive reasoning, the analysis progresses from the whole situation to specific parts or features, while inductive reasoning requires an analysis of parts or details to formulate an overall concept.[10] A form of inductive reasoning is analogic reasoning, which involves determining the relationship between similar situations and generalizing it to a new situation.

Reasoning has also been divided into convergent and divergent thinking. Convergent thinking is the analysis of information around a main idea or central topic.[10] Divergent thinking relates to flexibility of thought and is the creative generation of alternate ideas or interpretations.[26]

Problem solving requires both convergent and divergent thinking. It is a multicomponent process and involves the following steps: recognizing and analyzing a problem, developing alternate solutions for solving the problem, evaluating the solutions, selecting the most appropriate solution, implementing the solution, and evaluating its effectiveness.[26,27]

Judgment is an integral part of problem solving. It involves forming an opinion or estimate and predicting the consequences of an action based on known information.[26] Judgment is involved in the selection of the most appropriate solution and the evaluation of its effectiveness. Social judgment has been defined as knowing what is appropriate and inappropriate and applying reasoning to social situations.[10] In patients with right hemisphere damage, problems in social judgment are affected also by pragmatic deficits.

Orientation

Figure 3–1 shows that orientation is not a basic cognitive process but rather results from the interaction of attention, memory, and perception as well as the higher cognitive processes. Orientation is the awareness of self in relation to person, place, situation, and time.[18] Orientation to person is knowing oneself as well as others. Place (or geographic) orientation[28] includes being aware of where one is in the environment, finding one's way in familiar and new environments, and identifying places on maps or floor plans. Burns, Halper, and Mogil[29] differentiated between passive and active orientation to place. Being aware of one's present location is passive orientation, while finding one's way in the environment is active orientation. Orientation to situation is the awareness of the present situation and the circumstances leading up to it. Orientation to time includes both telling time (passive orientation) and monitoring the passage of time (active orientation).

Patients with right hemisphere damage may have particular difficulty with place orientation because they fail to perceive environmental cues accurately. For example, a patient believed he was in a ship because he saw Lake Michigan out of his window. Some patients may have difficulty finding their rooms because they cannot remember their room number. Further, they may not see signs on their left side or the name on the left side of the door. With regard to orientation to situation, some patients with right hemisphere damage may not be aware of their illness or the extent of their disability. They may not know the time, date, day, or season and may not be able to use environmental cues to orient themselves to time (e.g., darkness for time of day or snow on the ground for season).

EFFECTIVE COMMUNICATION SKILLS

Effective communication is dependent on adequate phonological, syntactical, morphological, semantic, and pragmatic skills. Phonology is the rule system for the way in which the sounds of the language are pronounced and combined.[30] The rules for what the words of the language are and how they are formed is morphology, while syntax refers to how words are combined into meaningful sequences. Semantics is attaching meaning to words and sentences. "Pragmatics is the study of the relationships between language behavior and the contexts in which it is used."[31] Pragmatics determines the social appropriateness of the language behavior. According to Davis,[32] pragmatics comprises three contexts—extralinguistic, paralinguistic, and linguistic.

The extralinguistic context exists separate from the utterance itself. It includes external factors such as the setting and the participants, and internal factors such as emotional state and knowledge of the participants. The extralinguistic context may be reflected by nonverbal behaviors such as gestures, body posture and position, eye contact, and facial expressions.

The paralinguistic context includes the suprasegmental features of intonation and prosody that are used to convey emotions or to signal semantic interpretation or syntactic analysis. Rising pitch indicating a question or different stress patterns on words (such as re'cord or rec'ord) are examples of the use of prosody.

The linguistic context refers to the verbal behavior or discourse that is a string of connected speech units. There are different kinds of discourse including narrative, procedural, and conversational discourse. Narrative discourse is the generation of a series of events usually recounted in the first or third person (e.g., telling a memorable experience or retelling a story). Procedural discourse refers to describing the steps involved in completing a task (e.g., how to make a sandwich).

Conversational discourse refers to a cooperative exchange of information between two or more people. Skills required for effective conversation include the appropriate initiation of a conversation, introduction of a new topic, maintenance of a topic, and turn-taking skills. Effective conversation also relies heavily on the adequate comprehension and production of nonverbal behaviors. For example, a speaker uses eye contact to evaluate the listener's interest in the topic, to establish role dominance, and as a turn-taking signal.

An important aspect of discourse production is the use of cohesive ties to allow for a smooth and logical flow of discourse. There are several types of cohesive ties such as reference, substitution, ellipsis, conjunction, and lexical cohesion.[33] The most common of these is reference, which is the use of pronouns, demonstratives (this/that), or comparatives to refer to previously mentioned items. Cohesive ties facilitate more organized discourse. When discourse is organized, information is ordered logically (e.g., temporally or procedurally around a main theme).

The patient with right hemisphere stroke may have difficulty interpreting the facial expression and body posture of a conversational partner and, therefore, may not understand the intent of the message. In addition, he or she may not understand or use conversational turn-taking signals, such as changes in intonation or gestures that indicate the end of a turn. Topic initiation and maintenance may be impaired, so the patient may not initiate appropriate topics for conversation or may digress from the topic being discussed. Some patients may provide too much information and are considered verbose, while other patients may provide insufficient details.[34-40]

INTERRELATIONSHIPS AMONG THE PROCESSES

In all individuals, the basic cognitive processes of attention, memory, and perception, and the higher-level cognitive processes of organization, reasoning, and problem solving/judgment are interrelated. Figure 3–1 shows some of the major interactions. The intent is not to specify every interaction but to highlight those that are important for understanding and managing cognitive-communication problems in right hemisphere damaged patients.

Focused, sustained, and selective attention allows individuals to filter out irrelevant sensory stimuli and attend to relevant stimuli long enough to process them perceptually and attach meaning to them. Once information has been processed perceptually, it is easier for an individual to sustain attention to it so that higher-level cognitive processing (e.g., reasoning) can occur.

For effective attention to an activity, the task requirements and the specific content must be held in working memory. Conversely, all levels of attention are important for maximizing successful encoding to or retrieval from memory. The accurate perceptual interpretation of sensory information is essential for the accurate encoding of information. The formation of meaningful perceptions is dependent on comparing present perceptions to those stored in memory. Organization, reasoning, and problem solving/judgment are highly interrelated, and most activities require all three of these processes.

In order to organize, reason, and problem solve, one needs to attend to, perceive, and remember the information necessary for the task. Attention, memory, and perception are facilitated by improved organization, reasoning, and problem solving.

In this framework, orientation is not considered a basic cognitive process, but rather requires the integrity of the other processes described previously. For example, memory (encoding, storage, and retrieval) for new information is important to orientation to place. Attention to and perception of environmental cues also facilitate orientation to place. Organization, more specifically categorization of the environmental cues, together with problem solving and reasoning strategies is essential for finding one's way around the environment.

Communicative interactions cannot occur unless the individual attends to, perceives, and remembers the verbal message and the subtle, nonverbal signals given by others. Ability to sequence ideas and events facilitates the production of meaningful, well-ordered, and logical discourse. Word choice and socially appropriate language behavior depends on the individual's analysis and judgment of the participants and the situation.

CONCLUSION

Effective communication skills are dependent on the integrity of the cognitive processes described previously. Communication skills in the patient with right hemisphere damage are less effective because of deficits in the underlying basic cognitive processes of attention, perception, and memory, and/or the higher-level cognitive processes of organization, reasoning, and problem solving/judgment. The clinical implications for diagnosis and treatment presented in the following chapters are based on this framework.

REFERENCES

1. Cummings JL. Hemispheric specialization: A history of current concepts. In: Burns MS, Halper AS, Mogil SI, eds. *Clinical Management of Right Hemisphere Dysfunction.* 1st ed. Gaithersburg, Md: Aspen Publishers, Inc; 1985:1–5.
2. Joanette Y, Goulet P. Right hemisphere and verbal communication: conceptual, methodological, and clinical issues. *Clin Aphasiology.* 1994;22:1–23.
3. Burns MS. Language without communication: The pragmatics of right hemisphere damage. In: Burns MS, Halper AS, Mogil SI, eds. *Clinical Management of Right Hemisphere Dysfunction.* 1st ed. Gaithersburg, Md: Aspen Publishers, Inc; 1985:17–28.
4. Joanette Y, Goulet P, Hannequin D. *Right Hemisphere and Verbal Communication.* New York, NY: Springer-Verlag; 1990.
5. Myers PS. Communication disorders associated with right-hemisphere brain damage. In: R. Chapey, ed. *Language Intervention Strategies in Adult Aphasia.* 3rd ed. Baltimore, Md: Williams & Wilkins; 1994:514–534.
6. Myers PS, Mackisack EL. Right hemisphere syndrome. In: LaPointe LL, ed. *Aphasia and Related Neurogenic Language Disorders.* New York, NY: Thieme Medical Publishers; 1990:177–195.
7. Tompkins CA. *Right Hemisphere Communication Disorders: Theory and Management.* San Diego, Calif: Singular Publishing Group, Inc; 1995.
8. American Speech-Language-Hearing Association, Subcommittee on Language. The role of speech-language pathologists in the habilitation and rehabilitation of cognitively impaired adults: A report of the subcommittee on language. *ASHA.* 1987;29:53–55.
9. Sohlberg MM, Mateer C. Effectiveness of an attention training program. *J Clin and Exper Neuropsychol.* 1987; 9:117–130.
10. Sohlberg MM, Mateer C. *Introduction to Cognitive Rehabilitation.* New York, NY: Guilford Press; 1989.
11. Mesulam, MM. Attention, confusional states and neglect. In: Mesulam MM, ed. *Principles of Behavioral Neurology.* Philadelphia, Pa: FA Davis Co; 1985:125–168.
12. Rapcsak SZ, Verfaellie M, Fleet WS, Heilman KM. Selective attention in hemispatial neglect. *Arch Neurol.* 1989;46:178–182.
13. Baddeley AD. Memory theory and memory therapy. In: Wilson BA, Moffat N, eds. *Clinical Management of Memory Problems.* Gaithersburg, Md: Aspen Publishers, Inc; 1984:5–27.
14. Signoret JL. Memory and amnesia. In: Mesulam MM, ed. *Principles of Behavioral Neurology.* Philadelphia, Pa: FA Davis Co; 1985:169–192.
15. Craik F, Lockhart R. Levels of processing: A framework for memory research. *J Verbal Learning and Verbal Behav.* 1972;11:671–684.
16. Baddeley AD, Hitch GJ. Working memory. In: Bower GA, ed. *The Psychology of Learning and Motivation: Advances in Research and Theory.* New York, NY: Academic Press, Inc; 1974:47–90.
17. Tompkins CA, Bloise CGR, Timko ML, Baumgartner A. Working memory and inference revision in brain-damaged and normally aging adults. *J Speech and Hearing Research.* 1994;35:626–637.
18. Lezak M. *Neuropsychological Assessment.* 2nd ed. New York, NY: Oxford University Press; 1983.
19. McCarthy RA, Warrington EK. *Cognitive Neuropsychology: A Clinical Introduction.* New York, NY: Academic Press, Inc; 1990.
20. Bihrle AM, Brownell HH, Powelson JA, Gardner H. Comprehension of humorous and non-humorous materials by left and right brain-damaged patients. *Brain and Cognition.* 1986;5:399–411.
21. Brownell HH, Michel D, Powelson J, Gardner H. Surprise but not coherence: Sensitivity to verbal humor in right-hemisphere patients. *Brain and Language.* 1983; 18:20–27.
22. Hier DB, Kaplan J. Verbal comprehension deficits after right hemisphere damage. *Applied Psycholinguistics.* 1980;1:279–294.
23. Foldi NS. Appreciation of pragmatic interpretation of indirect commands: Comparison of right and left hemisphere brain-damaged patients. *Brain and Language.* 1987;31:88–108.
24. Hirst W, LeDoux J, Stein S. Constraints on the processing of indirect speech acts: Evidence from aphasiology. *Brain and Language.* 1984;23:26–33.
25. Weylman ST, Brownell HH, Roman M, Gardner H. Appreciation of indirect requests by left- and right-brain-damaged patients: The effects of verbal context and conventionality of wording. *Brain and Language.* 1989;36: 580–591.
26. Szekeres SF, Ylvisaker M, Cohen SB. A framework for cognitive rehabilitation therapy. In: Ylvisaker M, Gobble EMR, eds. *Community Re-entry for Head Injured Adults.* Boston, Mass: College-Hill Press; 1987:87–136.
27. Luria AR. *Human Brain and Psychological Processes.* New York, NY: Harper & Row; 1966.
28. Strub RI, Black FW. *The Mental Status Examination in Neurology.* Philadelphia, Pa: FA Davis Co; 1977.
29. Burns MS, Halper AS, Mogil SI. Diagnosis of communication problems in right hemisphere damage. In: Burns MS, Halper AS, Mogil SI, eds. *Clinical Management of Right Hemisphere Dysfunction.* 1st ed. Gaithersburg, Md: Aspen Publishers, Inc; 1985:29–56.

30. Bloom L, Lahey M. *Language Development and Language Disorders.* New York, NY: John Wiley & Sons, Inc; 1978.
31. Davis GA, Wilcox MJ. *Adult Aphasia Rehabilitation: Applied Pragmatics.* San Diego, Calif: College-Hill Press; 1985.
32. Davis GA. Pragmatics and treatment. In: Chapey R, ed. *Language Intervention Strategies in Adult Aphasia.* 2nd ed. Baltimore, Md: Williams & Wilkins; 1986.
33. Halliday MAK, Hasan R. *Cohesion in English.* London: Longman; 1976.
34. Cherney LR, Canter GJ. Informational content in the discourse of patients with probable Alzheimer's disease and patients with right brain damage. *Clin Aphasiology.* 1993;21:123–134.
35. Joanette Y, Goulet P. Narrative discourse in right-brain-damaged right-handers. In: Joanette Y, Brownell HH, eds. *Discourse Ability and Brain Damage: Theoretical and Empirical Perspectives.* New York, NY: Springer-Verlag; 1990:131–153.
36. Kennedy M, Strand E, Burton W, Peterson C. Analysis of first-encounter conversations of right-hemisphere-damaged adults. *Clin Aphasiology.* 1994;22:67–80.
37. Myers PS. Narrative expressive deficits associated with right-hemisphere brain damage. In: Brownell HH, Joanette Y, eds. *Narrative Discourse in Neurologically Impaired and Normal Aging Adults.* San Diego, Calif: Singular Publishing Group, Inc; 1993:279–296.
38. Sheratt SM, Penn C. Discourse in a right-hemisphere brain damaged subject. *Aphasiology.* 1990;4:539–560.
39. Trupe EH, Hillis A. Paucity vs. verbosity: Another analysis of right hemisphere communication deficits. In: Brookshire RH, ed. *Clinical Aphasiology Conference Proceedings.* Minneapolis, Minn: BRK Publishers; 1985.
40. Uryase D, Duffy RJ, Liles BZ. Analysis and description of narrative discourse in right-hemisphere-damaged adults: A comparison with neurologically normal and left-hemisphere-damaged aphasic adults. *Clin Aphasiology.* 1990;19:125–137.

Chapter 4

RIC Evaluation of Communication Problems in Right Hemisphere Dysfunction-Revised (RICE-R): Statistical Background

Leora Reiff Cherney, Anita S. Halper,
Allen W. Heinemann, and Patrick Semik

INTRODUCTION

The Rehabilitation Institute of Chicago Evaluation of Communication Problems in Right Hemisphere Dysfunction (RICE)[1] was specifically designed to focus on those sequelae of right hemisphere damage known to be clinically important to the rehabilitative process. The subtests that were included in the RICE were based on current knowledge and clinical expertise at the time. The RICE consisted of the following subtests:

- Behavioral Observation Profile
- Visual Scanning and Tracking
- Assessment and Analysis of Writing
- Rating Scale of Pragmatic Communication Skills
- Metaphorical Language Test

When the test was developed, there was no other evaluation tool available to assess cognitive-communicative problems in patients with right hemisphere damage. Clinicians had depended on their informal observations and used tests designed for aphasia and other neurogenic communication disorders.

The RICE rating scales were developed to assist clinicians in providing structure to their informal observations and a measure for posttreatment comparison. Values were assigned according to the degree to which the patient deviated from a general standard of adequacy rather than normalcy. The standard of adequacy was chosen to permit the clinician to consider individual differences in cognitive style and evaluate each person relative to their premorbid characteristics, rather than comparing performance to a statistical norm. This method was important for evaluating such behaviors as communicative competence, because communication style is known to vary by socioeconomic class, sex, and age.

The authors gratefully acknowledge the assistance provided by Benjamin D. Wright, PhD, Professor, Department of Education, University of Chicago, Chicago, Illinois. His expertise in the use of the Rasch Analysis was invaluable. We also extend our thanks to the Speech-Language Pathologists in the Department of Communicative Disorders at the Rehabilitation Institute of Chicago for their assistance in testing patients with right hemisphere stroke.

This chapter addresses the further development of the RICE and provides data on its reliability and validity that were collected as part of the standardization process that led to the development of the RICE-Revised (RICE-R).

PHASE 1: ESTABLISHING INTERNAL CONSISTENCY OF THE ITEMS

The medical records of 65 consecutively admitted adult patients with unilateral right hemisphere stroke were reviewed to obtain the RICE test scores. All subjects met the following basic criteria: right handed, fluent speakers of English, at least an eighth-grade education, and hearing within normal limits for conversational speech. The age of the subjects ranged from 30 to 84 years (Mean = 61.7, SD = 14.4) and their education ranged from 8 to 20 years (Mean = 13.6, SD = 4.0). Stroke type included 45 subjects with a thrombosis, 19 with a hemorrhage, and 1 with an embolism. The group was heterogeneous in terms of site of lesion, which is presented in Table 4–1.

Table 4–1 Right Hemisphere Stroke Subjects: Site of Lesion (Phase 1)

Site of Lesion	Number	Percent
Frontal	7	10.8
Parietal	7	10.8
Temporal	3	4.6
Occipital	3	4.6
Frontoparietal	6	9.2
Temporoparietal	5	7.7
Occipitoparietal	3	4.6
Frontal-temporal-parietal	4	6.2
Basal ganglia—internal capsule	9	13.8
Anterior cerebral artery	2	3.1
Middle cerebral artery	7	10.8
Posterior cerebral artery	1	1.5
Thalamus	2	3.1
Other—records not available	6	9.2
Total	**65**	**100%**

Internal consistency was measured using coefficient alpha (Cronbach alpha).[2] Cronbach alpha ranges from 0 to 1, where a value of 0 indicates no internal consistency and a value of 1 indicates perfect internal consistency. It indicates the extent to which the items correlate with each other and form a coherent indicator of a single construct. Table 4–2 shows the alphas of the RICE subtests. In general, high inter-item consistency was obtained on all subtests except for Assessment and Analysis of Writing. Based on the results of this analysis and feedback by clinicians regarding the ease of administration and scoring, modifications were made to the RICE. The following are the modifications made to the original RICE (1985) based on the internal consistency measures presented in Table 4–2.

Behavioral Observation Profile

The Behavioral Observation Profile was streamlined by omitting from this subtest those items that are also included in the Rating Scale of Pragmatic Communication Skills. These items included eye contact, facial expression, intonation, and topic maintenance. One additional item, memory for daily events, was added to the subtest. No measure of memory was included in the original RICE.

Rating Scale of Pragmatic Communication Skills

The item that measured verbosity was changed to measure response length, to account for both verbosity and reduced output. The two items that measured organization of a narrative were removed. However, completeness of a narrative was retained as a separate item, which is based on the Story Retelling-Immediate Subtest of the *Arizona Battery for Communication Disorders of Dementia*.[3] The task has a maximum of 17 information units.

Visual Scanning and Tracking

A practice task with specific directions to be given to the patient has been added. The layout of

Table 4–2 Internal Consistency of the RICE

Subtest	N	Maximum Score Possible	Mean	SD	Standard Error	Alpha
Behavioral Observation Profile	65	45	31.32	8.29	1.03	.90
Rating Scale of Pragmatic Communication Skills	65	60	42.05	10.45	1.30	.89
Visual Scanning and Tracking	25	123	41.08	37.92	7.58	.76
Assessment and Analysis of Writing	47	55	46.79	4.97	0.73	.57
Metaphorical Language Test	53	10	4.34	2.62	0.36	.75

the subtest has been improved, so that it includes one scanning task per page. In addition, the instructions for scoring have been clarified. The error score is defined as the number of omissions of the target letter plus the number of nontarget letters selected. Measurement of time is specified in seconds.

Assessment and Analysis of Writing

This subtest was divided into two parts: one part for the patient who could copy and write words to dictation, and the other part for the patient who could complete a spontaneous writing sample of at least 50 words. The visuospatial disorganization item was divided into two items, one for lines progressing on a diagonal and one for superimposed letters. Two items, incomplete sentences and ungrammatic sentences, were combined. Finally, three items were removed: phonetically based and visually based spelling errors were omitted because of difficulty in determining the cause of the spelling errors; omission of strokes was removed because many normal subjects omit strokes.

Metaphorical Language Test

Five additional items were added to the Metaphorical Language Test. The scoring system was modified to include a "no response" category, and point values were assigned to each category as follows: normal abstract interpretation is worth 2 points; a partially correct response is worth 1 point; and all other responses are worth 0 points.

PHASE 2: STANDARDIZATION OF THE RICE-R

Subjects

The modified RICE was administered to 40 subjects with unilateral right hemisphere stroke and 36 normal subjects. All subjects were right handed, fluent speakers of English, with at least an eighth-grade education. Subjects displayed adequate hearing acuity for conversation and corrected vision for reading average-size print. No history of alcohol or drug abuse or history of previous neurologic or psychiatric disorders was evident. In addition, the normal subjects all passed the Mini-Mental State Examination, with the exception of one person. (This subject achieved a score one point below the cutoff of 25; the subject lost five points because he was unable to spell WORLD backward.) Characteristics of the subjects are provided in Table 4–3. No significant differences in age and education were present between the subjects with right hemisphere stroke and normal control subjects.

The subjects with right hemisphere stroke all had single lesions as confirmed by the computed tomography (CT) scan or by clinical examination. Length of time since onset for 39 of the 40 subjects ranged from 5 days to 269 days, with a mean of 73 days. Length of time since onset for the 40th patient was 687 days. Type of stroke varied: the majority of patients (25 of the 40 subjects) presented with thrombotic stroke, 11 presented with hemorrhagic stroke, and 3 presented with an embolic stroke. In one subject, type of stroke and site

Table 4–3 Phase 2: Demographic Characteristics of Subjects in the Standardization Sample

Variable	Normal Subjects	Subjects with Right Hemisphere Damage	Significance Testing
Sex			
Male	N = 10	N = 18	
Female	N = 26	N = 22	
Age			
Range	46–85	30–89	
Mean	59.40	60.70	t = 0.44; p = .66
SD	10.24	15.15	
Education			
Range	11–18	12–18	
Mean	14.55	13.67	t = –1.91; p = .06
SD	1.95	2.06	

of lesion were not clear but the patient had right symmetric periventricular area of decreased attenuation on a CT scan and demonstrated signs of a right hemisphere stroke on clinical examination. Table 4–4 presents site of lesion information for the subjects with right hemisphere stroke.

Procedures

The RICE was administered to patients with right hemisphere damage and scored by the patients' speech-language pathologists. The testing was videotaped, and tests were scored by both investigators. Administration of the RICE and the Mini-Mental State Examination to control subjects was completed and videotaped by a trained research assistant. Subsequently, both investigators scored these tests.

Reliability

Interrater reliability for each scale was obtained between two trained (investigators) raters and then between a trained and untrained (clinician) rater for the patients with right hemisphere damage. All correlations for trained/trained raters and trained/untrained raters were statistically significant (p < .01). However, as expected, interrater reliability was lower when one of the raters was not trained. Correlations dropped from .96 to .71 for the Behavioral Observation Profile, from .98 to .52 for the Rating Scale of Pragmatic Communication Skills, from 1.00 to .99 for errors and 1.00 to .98

Table 4–4 Right Hemisphere Stroke Subjects: Site of Lesion (Phase 2)

Site of Lesion	Number	Percent
Frontal	4	10.0
Parietal	4	10.0
Temporal	2	5.0
Occipital	1	2.5
Frontoparietal	3	7.5
Temporoparietal	6	15.0
Frontal-temporal-parietal	3	7.5
Basal ganglia—internal capsule	7	17.5
Anterior cerebral artery	1	2.5
Middle cerebral artery	4	10.0
Posterior cerebral artery	2	5.0
Normal CT scan	1	2.5
Other—records not available	2	5.0
Total	**40**	**100%**

for time on Visual Scanning and Tracking, from .99 to .96 for Assessment and Analysis of Writing, and from .99 to .78 for the Metaphorical Language Test. These results suggest that training is necessary to increase reliable use of the rating scale, particularly pragmatics. All of the data presented in this chapter are based on the ratings of a trained rater.

Validity

This section addresses issues related to the validity of the modified RICE.

Rasch Analysis

Construct validity refers to whether the test measures the characteristics it purports to measure. Items should cohere to form a single construct, and within that construct they should be ordered in difficulty according to clinical experience.[4] Rasch analysis[5] provides a means of estimating item difficulty, estimating item fit to the underlying construct, and transforming ordinal observations to linear measures for each person.[6]

The Rasch analysis was initially used for the three rating scales and metaphorical language. Based on the initial results, it was determined that a four-category scale works better than a five-category scale for the Behavioral Observation Profile and the Rating Scale of Pragmatic Communication Skills. The Assessment and Analysis of Writing yielded the best fit or validity statistics when a combination of a two-point, three-point, and five-point scale was used for specific items. On the Metaphorical Language Test, it was determined that scoring on a three-category scale maximized the range of ability measured in a consistent manner.

Table 4–5 compares the fit statistics for the five-category scales in the modified RICE and the revised four-category scales. The useful range of mean-square fit statistics is 0.7 to 1.3. This is the range that protects patient measures from problems due to item misfit. Values near 1.0 indicate satisfactory fit; values below 0.7 or above 1.3 indicate a misfit and threaten valid measurement. Values above 1.3 indicate that items contain an excess

Table 4–5 Rasch Analysis Results

Subtest	Five-Point Scale		Revised Scale	
	ISR*	PS†	ISR*	PS†
Behavioral Observation Profile	.91	3.03	.90	3.01
Rating Scale of Pragmatic Communication Skills	.89	2.58	.89	2.66
Assessment and Analysis of Writing	.90	.53	.80	1.07

* ISR = Item separation reliability
† PS = Person separation

of information (noise) and lack coherence between ratings on the item and the overall severity of the patient. Values less than 0.7 indicate that the item provides little independent information as to patient status. Acceptable person separation typically exceeds 2.0, which means two strata can be distinguished. On the revised scales, it can be seen that item separation reliability falls within the acceptable range for all subtests. Person separation exceeds the acceptable cutoff for the Behavioral Observation Profile and Rating Scale of Pragmatic Communication Skills. While the person separation is still below the 2.0 cutoff on the revised Assessment and Analysis of Writing, it is substantially better than the original scale. Item separation reliability is in the acceptable range, thus supporting use of the revised writing scale.

BIGSTEPS[6] also provides a measure of how well each item correlates with the total score. The point-biserial correlation provides a traditional measure of validity. Values of .7 to 1.0 are considered to be acceptable. Tables 4–6 to 4–9 provide the point-biserial correlations for each item in the Behavioral Observation Profile, Rating Scale of Pragmatic Communication Skills, Assessment and Analysis of Writing, and Metaphorical Language Test. These tables also show the order of difficulty of each item within the scale and provide the in-fit and out-fit statistics (standard deviations of item difficulties, average mean squares of items, and typical standard error of items). Desirable in-fit and out-fit statistics have a mean of 0 and a standard deviation of 1. A Z standard error score greater than 2 indicates that an item is excessively noisy and contains excessive information.

Behavioral Observation Profile. Table 4–6 shows that the point-biserial correlations range from .72 to .85, indicating that each item correlates well with the total score for this subtest. Not surprising, orientation to person is the easiest item on the scale, and orientation to time is the most difficult. In-fit and out-fit mean squares are in the acceptable range for all items.

Rating Scale of Pragmatic Communication Skills. Table 4–7 shows that the point-biserial correlations range from .70 to .85 for seven areas (facial expression, intonation, gestures and proxemics, conversational initiation, eye contact, turn taking, and topic maintenance), indicating that each of these items correlates well with the total score for this subtest. Presupposition and referencing skills have moderate correlations with the total score for this subtest. This can be attributed to the fact that conversational speech about everyday topics may not reveal deficits in these areas. It is recommended that clinicians use conversation about less familiar, more abstract topics to probe for deficits in presupposition and referencing. The low point-biserial correlation for response length (.58) and large mean square in-fit (1.59) reflect the fact that this item incorporates two aspects of response length—verbosity or short utterances. Overall, the nonverbal areas of facial expression and intonation were the most difficult items on the rating scale, while topic maintenance and turn taking were the easiest for the patients with right hemisphere damage. In-fit and out-fit mean squares are in the acceptable range for all items.

Narrative Discourse—Completeness. Because the test contains only one item in this area, Rasch analysis cannot be used. Instead, data were analyzed using the *t*-test and examining the frequency distribution of scores obtained from control subjects and patients with right hemisphere damage. See section entitled "Determining Severity Levels" for details.

Assessment and Analysis of Writing. Table 4–8 shows that the in-fit and out-fit statistics are within the acceptable range for all items. The point-biserial correlations range from .02 to .64. Clinically, effective writing requires multiple skills, including such dimensions as visuospatial organization, linguistic organization, and relevancy of content. Therefore, as expected, many of the individual items on this subject do not correlate highly with the total writing subtest score. The table shows that the most difficult items for patients with right hemisphere damage are related to left-side neglect, while the easiest items are related to

Table 4–6 Point-Biserial Correlations and In-Fit and Out-Fit Statistics: Behavioral Observation Profile

Subtest	Point Biserial Correlation	Measure	Error	In-Fit Mean Square	In-Fit Z-Standard Error	Out-Fit Mean Square	Out-Fit Z-Standard Error
Orientation to time	.80	1.56	.34	1.30	1.30	1.25	1.00
Awareness of illness	.83	0.67	.34	0.66	−1.70	0.66	−1.70
Orientation to place	.77	0.56	.34	1.06	0.30	1.10	0.40
Memory for daily events	.81	0.33	.34	0.73	−1.30	0.77	−1.10
Attention	.72	−1.00	.36	1.27	1.00	1.68	1.70
Orientation to person	.85	−2.11	.39	0.70	−1.30	0.53	−1.00

Table 4–7 Point-Biserial Correlations and In-Fit and Out-Fit Statistics: Rating Scale of Pragmatic Communication Skills

Subtest	Point Biserial Correlation	Measure	Error	In-Fit		Out-Fit	
				Mean Square	Z-Standard Error	Mean Square	Z-Standard Error
Facial expression	.73	1.39	.24	1.07	0.30	1.02	0.10
Intonation	.72	1.09	.24	1.24	1.00	1.15	0.60
Gestures and proxemics	.84	0.27	.25	0.81	−0.90	0.66	−1.50
Conversational initiation	.85	0.27	.25	0.61	−2.10	0.53	−2.20
Response length	.58	0.21	.25	1.59	2.30	1.70	2.10
Presupposition	.65	−0.12	.26	1.05	0.20	0.89	−0.40
Eye contact	.74	−0.23	.25	1.05	0.20	0.84	−0.50
Referencing skills	.64	−0.39	.26	1.12	0.50	1.31	0.80
Turn taking	.70	−0.84	.27	0.81	−0.80	0.73	−0.70
Topic maintenance	.77	−1.64	.30	0.52	−2.20	−0.48	−1.10

Table 4–8 Point-Biserial Correlations and In-Fit and Out-Fit Statistics: Assessment and Analysis of Writing

Subtest	Point Biserial Correlation	Measure	Error	In-Fit		Out-Fit	
				Mean Square	Z-Standard Error	Mean Square	Z-Standard Error
Presence of left-sided neglect	.48	1.34	.34	0.81	−1.30	0.77	−1.10
Degree of left-sided neglect	.36	0.83	.17	1.14	0.70	1.04	0.20
Run-on sentences	.45	0.47	.23	0.90	−0.50	1.25	0.60
Incomplete/ungrammatical sentences	.52	0.31	.23	0.79	−1.10	1.00	0.00
Visuospatial disorganization—lines	.24	0.14	.36	1.16	0.90	1.09	0.30
Ambiguous sentences	.64	−0.09	.25	0.71	−1.40	0.40	−1.60
Perseveration of strokes and/or letters	.23	−0.28	.39	1.21	1.00	0.93	−0.20
Omission of letters	.31	−0.98	.45	0.94	−0.20	1.42	0.70
Visuospatial disorganization—superimposed letters	.02	−1.74	.56	1.33	0.80	1.18	0.20

visuospatial disorganization (superimposed letters) and omission and perseveration of letters.

Metaphorical Language Test. Table 4–9 shows that the in-fit and out-fit statistics are within the acceptable range except for "a stitch in time saves nine" with an in-fit mean square of 1.34. The point biserial correlations range from .14 to .62. No item by itself has a high point-biserial correlation. The easiest items for patients with right hemisphere damage are "It's raining cats and dogs" and "Don't beat around the bush," and the most difficult items are "Your name will be mud" and "You cannot burn the candle at both ends." Clinically, it is important to include both easy and difficult items to assess the range of severity in this population. Therefore, this subtest can be administered to severely and mildly impaired patients.

While item separation reliability (.94) is good, person separation (1.73) falls below the acceptable cutoff of two logits. Further refinements will evaluate harder and easier items that should be included.

Significance Testing

Significance testing was conducted on the total scores achieved by both subject groups on each subtest of the RICE. Table 4–10 shows a significant difference between the two groups ($p < .001$) for each subtest.

Table 4–9 Point-Biserial Correlations and In-Fit and Out-Fit Statistics: Metaphorical Language Test

Subtest	Point Biserial Correlation	Measure	Error	In-Fit Mean Square	In-Fit Z-Standard Error	Out-Fit Mean Square	Out-Fit Z-Standard Error
Your name will be mud	.35	1.43	.18	1.22	1.40	1.16	0.70
You cannot burn the candle at both ends	.36	0.87	.17	0.90	−0.80	0.97	−0.20
A stitch in time saves nine	.31	0.73	.17	1.34	2.30	1.31	1.70
Read between the lines	.54	0.73	.17	0.97	−0.20	0.88	−0.70
It takes two to tango	.46	0.57	.17	1.02	0.10	0.99	0.00
Look before you leap	.40	0.40	.17	0.93	−0.50	0.93	−0.40
Two heads are better than one	.58	0.14	.17	0.69	−2.40	0.80	−1.10
Save it for a rainy day	.42	0.05	.17	1.09	0.60	1.08	0.40
He is my right hand	.48	−0.08	.18	1.03	0.20	1.01	0.00
Nothing ventured, nothing gained	.62	−0.14	.18	0.85	−1.00	0.71	−1.40
Look down one's nose at	.54	−0.48	.19	0.96	−0.20	0.81	−0.70
He's a chip off the old block	.35	−0.52	.19	1.16	0.90	1.31	1.00
The apple of my eye	.54	−0.75	.20	0.85	−0.90	0.80	−0.70
Don't beat around the bush	.32	−0.93	.22	1.09	0.40	0.91	−0.30
It's raining cats and dogs	.14	−2.01	.33	1.29	0.70	1.31	0.50

Determining Severity Levels

Cutoff scores for differentiating normal subjects from patients with right hemisphere damage were determined separately for each subtest. These were derived from the frequency distribution of scores achieved by each group of subjects. The criterion was used to minimize the number of misclassifications in each group. The percentage of normal subjects and patients with right hemisphere damage who were correctly classified in our sample using these cutoff points is discussed below.

Guidelines for severity levels for each subtest were determined by dividing approximately into thirds the distribution of patients' scores below the cutoff point. However, the clinician should consider the pattern of performance and implications of deficits within each subtest on everyday functioning when determining the overall severity of a patient's deficits. Table 4–11 shows the suggested range of scores for mild, moderate, and severe severity levels.

Behavioral Observation Profile. A cutoff score of 23 correctly classified 100% of the normal subjects and 80% of the patients with right hemisphere damage.

Rating Scale of Pragmatic Communication Skills. A cutoff score of 38 correctly classified 100% of the normal subjects and 80% of the patients with right hemisphere damage.

Narrative Discourse—Completeness. A cutoff score of 15 correctly classified 66% of the normal subjects and 69% of the patients with right hemisphere damage. This means that approximately one third of the normal subjects scored poorly, and approximately one third of the patients with right hemisphere damage scored as well as the normal subjects. These results are not surprising, since normal subjects vary in their ability to recall details auditorily, and some patients with right hemisphere damage perform within normal limits on verbal tasks.

Visual Scanning and Tracking. A cutoff score of 5 errors correctly classified 94% of the normal subjects and 86% of the patients with right hemisphere damage. The cutoff score of 210 seconds to complete all tasks correctly classified 86% of normal subjects and 94% of patients with right hemisphere damage. The clinician should keep in mind that some patients may perform above the cutoff point in either accuracy or time.

Assessment and Analysis of Writing. A cutoff score of 22 correctly classified 100% of the normal subjects and 82% of the patients with right hemisphere damage.

Metaphorical Language Test. Metaphorical language cutoff points were determined some-

Table 4–10 Comparison of Subjects with Right Hemisphere Damage and Normal Controls

Subtest	Total Possible Score	Right Hemisphere Damage		Controls		p
		Mean	SD	Mean	SD	
Behavioral Observation Profile	24	17.45	5.03	24.00	0	<.001
Rating Scale of Pragmatic Communication Skills	40	29.00	7.73	39.80	0.53	<.001
Visual Scanning and Tracking						
• Accuracy (No. of errors)	97 target items 340 nontarget items	52.61	37.43	1.47	2.34	<.001
• Rate (in seconds)	No maximum time	453.08	262.12	165.11	38.43	<.001
Assessment and Analysis of Writing	24	18.29	3.84	23.54	0.66	<.001
Metaphorical Language Test	30	16.37	6.10	22.50	4.79	<.001

Table 4–11 Guidelines for Assigning Severity Levels from Scores

Subtest	Maximum Score Possible	Normal Range	Severity Level		
			Mild	Moderate	Severe
Behavioral Observation Profile	24	23–24	19–22	14–18	13
Rating Scale of Pragmatic Communication Skills	40	38–40	30–37	25–29	24
Visual Scanning and Tracking					
• Errors	437	5	6–16	17–70	71
• Time	N/A	210 seconds	211–390	391–549	550 seconds
Assessment and Analysis of Writing	24	22–24	19–21	16–18	15
Metaphorical Language Test	30	High Average: 28–30 Average: 20–27	17–19	13–16	12

what differently since there was a wide range of scores for the normal group. Scores falling in the 20th to 80th percentile of the normal group were considered to be average. This percentile range represents approximately one standard deviation above and below the mean test scores in the normal distribution. Scores falling above the 80th percentile (raw scores of 28–30) were considered above average. Scores falling below the 20th percentile (19 and below) were considered to be in the deficit range. Using a cutoff score of 20, 78% of the normal subjects and 70% of the patients with right hemisphere damage were correctly classified.

CONCLUSION

The process of establishing reliability and validity of the RICE-R has involved several phases that have focused on establishing internal consistency of the items, revising the original RICE, and standardizing the RICE-R. The subject sample included individuals with right hemisphere damage and normal controls. This sample has yielded information regarding the performance of normal subjects, which provides guidelines for identifying impaired performance. The RICE-R is presented in Appendix A, and guidelines for its administration are presented in Appendix B.

REFERENCES

1. Burns MS, Halper AS, Mogil SI. RIC evaluation of communication problems in right hemisphere dysfunction. In: Burns MS, Halper AS, Mogil SI, eds. *Clinical Management of Right Hemisphere Dysfunction*. 1st ed. Gaithersburg, Md: Aspen Publishers, Inc; 1985.

2. Cronbach LT. Coefficient alpha and the internal structure of tests. *Psychometrika*. 1951;16:295–335.

3. Bayles KA, Tomoeda CK. *Arizona Battery for Communication Disorders of Dementia*. Tucson, Ariz: Canyonland Publishing, Inc; 1991.

4. Wright BD, Stone MH. *Best Test Design: Rasch Measurement*. Chicago, Ill: MESA Press; 1979.

5. Rasch G. *Probabilistic Models for Some Intelligence and Attainment Tests*. Chicago, Ill: University of Chicago Press; 1980 (Originally published in 1960).

6. Linacre JM. *BIGSTEPS for PC Compatibles*. Chicago, Ill: MESA Press; 1995.

Chapter 5

Tests for Evaluating Cognitive-Communicative Skills in Patients with Right Hemisphere Damage

Anita S. Halper and Leora Reiff Cherney

This chapter presents an annotated list of formal standardized tests (see Table 5–1). While this list is not exhaustive, it includes those tests or selected subtests that we have found to be most valuable for assessing the cognitive-communicative skills of the adult with right brain damage. All of the tests are commercially available and readily accessible to speech-language pathologists. Furthermore, the tests evaluate those areas known to be impaired in this population that impact on communication. The list indicates those processes that are primarily assessed by the test, although several other processes may be required to perform the task. The speech-language pathologist should consider these other processes in analyzing the reasons for the patient's difficulty with the task. For example, a patient may have problems performing a visually presented reasoning task because of unilateral left neglect rather than reasoning problems. Failure could also be the result of visual perceptual problems with the stimuli not being perceived correctly. Similarly, a reasoning task presented auditorily may be difficult due to memory deficits.

Also included in the list of tests are two test batteries designed specifically for use with patients with right hemisphere damage. The Mini Inventory of Right Brain Injury by Pimental and Kingsbury was developed in 1989. It serves as a screening tool to differentiate individuals with right hemisphere damage and normal adults. The Right Hemisphere Language Battery, Second Edition, by Bryan was revised in 1995. It was designed to assess the presence of language disorders in patients with right hemisphere damage. This battery includes several subtests that focus on comprehension of abstract material such as humor and metaphors.

In the current health care climate, evaluations must be completed in a very short period of time—often not more than one or two sessions. Therefore, the speech-language pathologist cannot perform a comprehensive evaluation that assesses all cognitive-communicative areas. Rather, the clinician must selectively evaluate only those areas of highest priority. In determining priorities, the speech-language pathologist must consider the severity level of the patient; the patient's premorbid educational, vocational, and avocational status; and, most importantly, discharge placement and patient/family goals (e.g., home, nursing home, return to work or school). Other areas may be evaluated if and when changes in the patient's status, needs, and goals occur. In most instances, the clinician does not need to administer the complete test, but only subtests of the battery that are appropriate.

Table 5-1 Tests for Evaluating Cognitive-Communicative Skills in Patients with Right Hemispheric Damage

Test/Subtest	Attention	Memory	Perception	Orientation	Higher Cognitive Processes	Communication: Pragmatics (PR)/Semantics (S)
Behavioural Inattention Test (BIT), by B. Wilson, J. Cockburn, and P. Halligan (1987), Thames Valley Test Company. Available from: Northern Speech Services, Inc., 117 North Elm Street, PO Box 1247, Gaylord, MI 49735. Assesses unilateral visual neglect via six pencil-and-paper subtests and nine functional subtests.						
Line crossing—Assesses ability to cross out 36 one-inch-long lines distributed across the page.	X					
Letter cancellation—Assesses ability to cross out 40 stimulus letters (*E* and *R*) that are randomly distributed across five lines of letters.	X					
Star cancellation—Assesses ability to cross out 54 small stars scattered across a page that contains small stars and randomly distributed large stars, letters, and short words.	X					
Figure and shape copying—Assesses ability to copy three drawings (star, cube, daisy) and three geometric shapes.	X					
Line bisection—Assesses ability to bisect the center of three horizontal eight-inch lines.	X					

Tests for Evaluating Cognitive-Communicative Skills 43

		X
		X
		X
		X
		X
		X
		X
		X
		X
		X

Representational drawing—Assesses ability to draw three items spontaneously (clock face with numbers, person, butterfly).

Picture scanning—Assesses ability to identify items in a composite photograph.

Telephone dialing—Assesses ability to dial phone numbers that are presented on a card.

Menu reading—Assesses ability to read items on a menu.

Article reading—Assesses ability to read aloud a short, three-column article.

Telling and setting the time—Assesses ability to read the time from a digital and analog clock face and to set the time on the analog clock face.

Coin sorting—Assesses ability to identify coins arranged in three rows.

Address and sentence copying—Assesses ability to copy an address and a sentence.

Map navigation—Assesses ability to identify points on a simple map of a road system and move from one point to another.

Card sorting—Assesses ability to identify specific playing cards arranged in four rows.

This test is normed on 54 right hemisphere stroke subjects, 26 left hemisphere stroke subjects, and 50 controls. Mean score, standard deviation, and range of acceptable performance for the normal control group for each subtest are provided.

continues

Table 5–1 continued

Test/Subtest	Attention	Memory	Perception	Orientation	Higher Cognitive Processes	Communication: Pragmatics (PR)/ Semantics (S)
California Verbal Learning Test, by D.C. Delis, J.H. Kramer, E. Kaplan, and B.A. Ober (1987). Available from: The Psychological Corporation, 555 Academic Court, San Antonio, TX 78204.		X				
Assesses recall and recognition of word lists over a number of different trials.						
This test is normed on 104 males and 169 females 17 to 80 years of age. Raw scores can be expressed as a standard score that shows the number of standard deviations by which it deviates from the expected mean for that age and sex.						
Detroit Tests of Learning Aptitude–Adult, by D.D. Hammill and B.R. Bryant (1991). Available from: Pro-Ed, 8700 Shoal Creek Boulevard, Austin, TX 78758.					X	
Subtest II: Story Sequences—Assesses ability to sequence a series of cartoon-like pictures into a meaningful humorous story.						
Subtest III: Sentence Imitation—Assesses immediate recall of sentences of increasing length and complexity read aloud to the patient.	X	X				
Subtest IV: Reversed Letters—Assesses ability to write, in reverse order, a series of letters read aloud.	X	X				

Process Assessed

Tests for Evaluating Cognitive-Communicative Skills   45

Description	Col 1	Col 2	Col 3	Col 4
Subtest VI: Design Sequences—Assesses ability to arrange a series of cubes so as to reproduce a design sequence previously shown for five seconds.		X	X	
Subtest IX: Word Sequences—Assesses ability to recall a series of unrelated words read aloud.		X		
Subtest X: Design Reproduction—Assesses ability to reproduce figures from memory.		X		
Subtest XI: Symbolic Relations—Assesses ability to solve a visual problem involving geometric or line drawings.			X	
Subtest XII: Form Assembly—Assesses ability to create a whole figure by assembling its parts.				X
This test was normed on 1,254 subjects 16 to 79 years of age. Standard scores and percentile ranks are provided.				
Doors and People, by A. Baddeley, H. Emslie, and I. Nimmo-Smith (1995), Thames Valley Test Company. Available from: Northern Speech Services, Inc., 117 North Elm Street, PO Box 1247, Gaylord, MI 49735.				
Assesses visual and verbal recall and recognition via four subtests.				
Visual recognition—Assesses ability to memorize a series of colored photographs of doors and recognize each target door from a set of four doors.		X		X
Visual recall—Assesses ability to copy patterns and spontaneously draw them from memory over three learning trials; a delayed recall situation is included.		X		X

continues

Table 5–1 continued

Test/Subtest	Attention	Memory	Perception	Orientation	Higher Cognitive Processes	Communication: Pragmatics (PR)/ Semantics (S)
Verbal recognition—Assesses ability to memorize a series of names and recognize each target name from a set of four items.		X				
Verbal recall—Assesses ability to learn the names of four people over three learning trials; a delayed recall situation is included.		X				

The test is normed on 238 normal subjects and a preliminary sample of patients with Alzheimer's disease and patients with temporal lobectomies. It gives a single, age-scaled overall score, as well as separate measures of visual and verbal memory, recall and recognition, and rate of forgetting.

Mini Inventory of Right Brain Injury, by P.A. Pimental and N.A. Kingsbury (1989). Available from: Pro-Ed, 8700 Shoal Creek Boulevard, Austin, TX 78758.

Assesses visual processing, language processing, emotion and affect, and general behavior via a 27-item screening test designed specifically for patients with right hemisphere damage.

Tests for Evaluating Cognitive-Communicative Skills   47

continues

Visual processing—Screens visual scanning and tracking, finger gnosis, astereognosis, two-point discrimination, unilateral left neglect, oral reading, spontaneous writing, writing sentences to dictation, writing alternating letter sequences, serial 7s, and drawing a clock for a total of 21 points.

Language processing—Screens ability to express emotional tone of voice, understand humor, explain incongruities and absurdities, explain figurative language, and explain similarities for a total of 18 points.

Emotion and affect processing—Screens for flat affect for a total of 1 point.

General behavior and psychic integrity—Screens for impulsivity, distractibility, and ability to use eye contact for a total of 3 points.

This test is standardized on 30 right hemisphere injured patients and 30 normal controls. It provides a cutoff score that differentiates normal subjects from patients with right hemisphere damage.

The Right Hemisphere Language Battery, 2nd edition, by K.L. Bryan (1995). Available from: Whurr Publishers, Ltd., 19b Compton Terrace, London N1 2UN, England.

Assesses lexical-semantic processing, high-level language processing, and prosody via a test battery designed specifically for patients with right hemisphere damage.

Metaphor picture test—Assesses ability to understand metaphorical language; the subject is required to match an auditorily presented metaphor to one of four pictures.

Table 5-1 continued

Test/Subtest	Process Assessed					Communication: Pragmatics (PR)/ Semantics (S)
	Attention	Memory	Perception	Orientation	Higher Cognitive Processes	
Written metaphor test—Assesses ability to understand metaphorical language; the subject is required to match a metaphor incorporated into a sentence to one of three printed sentences.					X	
Comprehension of inferred meaning—Assesses ability to comprehend aspects of inferential meaning in a short, written paragraph.					X	
Appreciation of humor—Assesses ability to understand humor; the subject is required to select a punchline of a written joke from a choice of four.					X	
Lexical semantic test—Assesses ability to match a target word to one of five pictures.						X(S)
Production of emphatic stress—Assesses ability to complete sentences using stress on designated words.						X(PR)
Discourse analysis—Assesses conversation via a four-point rating scale that includes 15 parameters.						X(PR)

This test is standardized on 30 neurologically normal subjects, 40 right hemisphere damaged subjects, and 40 aphasic subjects. Means and standard deviations for these three groups are given.

The Rivermead Behavioural Memory Test, by B. Wilson, J. Cockburn, and A. Baddeley (1991), Thames Valley Test Company. Available from: Northern Speech Services, Inc., 117 North Elm Street, PO Box 1247, Gaylord, MI 49735.

Assesses everyday memory including remembering an appointment, remembering a belonging, picture recognition, immediate and delayed story recall, face recognition, remembering a short route, remembering to deliver a message, orientation, and remembering a name.

The test was normed on subjects 11 to 95 years of age. Two scores are available—a screening score based on a pass/fail grading of each item and a more detailed profile score. Both scores provide cutoff points for level of memory function (normal, poor memory, moderately impaired, severely impaired). Four parallel versions of the test are available.

Ross Information Processing Assessment, 2nd Edition (RIPA-2), by D. Ross-Swain (1995). Available from: Pro-Ed, 8700 Shoal Creek Boulevard, Austin, TX 78758.

I. Immediate Memory—Assesses immediate recall of numbers, words, and sentences of increasing length and complexity read aloud.

II. Recent Memory—Assesses recall of information related to the environment and daily activities.

III. Temporal Orientation (Recent Memory)—Assesses time orientation in relation to newly learned information.

IV. Temporal Orientation (Remote Memory)—Assesses remote memory of time concepts.

continues

Table 5–1 continued

Test/Subtest	Attention	Memory	Perception	Orientation	Higher Cognitive Processes	Communication: Pragmatics (PR)/ Semantics (S)
V. Spatial Orientation—Assesses recent and remote memory of spatial (place) orientation concepts.		X		X		
VI. Orientation to Environment—Assesses awareness and perception of the environment.		X		X		
VII. Recall of General Information—Assesses ability to recall general information in remote memory.		X				
VIII. Problem Solving and Abstract Reasoning—Assesses ability to problem solve and use reasoning strategies.					X	
IX. Organization—Assesses ability to name category members and recall a category name given specific category members.					X	X(S)
X. Auditory Processing and Retention—Assesses ability to comprehend yes/no questions containing temporal, spatial, and comparative information.					X	

This test was normed on 126 traumatically brain injured individuals. Therefore, the normative data cannot be used for patients with right hemisphere damage. However, instructions are given for scoring qualitatively using diacritical markings, for such responses as delayed, perseverative, irrelevant, and tangential.

Test of Everyday Attention, by I. Robertson, T. Ward, V. Ridgeway, and I. Nimmo-Smith (1994), Thames Valley Test Company. Available from: Northern Speech Services, Inc., 117 North Elm Street, PO Box 1247, Gaylord, MI 49735.

Assesses selective attention, sustained attention, and attentional switching capacities via eight subtests.

Map search—Assesses selective attention via ability to search for symbols on a colored map for a maximum of two minutes.

Elevator counting—Assesses sustained attention via ability to count a series of tape-presented tones simulating a situation in which an elevator's floor-indicator is not functioning.

Elevator counting with distraction—Assesses selective attention via ability to count a series of low tape-presented tones while ignoring high tones.

Visual elevator—Assesses alternating attention via ability to count up and down, simulating a situation for following the floors in an elevator from a visual cue.

Auditory elevator with reversal—Assesses alternating attention via ability to count up and down, simulating a situation of following the floors in an elevator from an auditory cue.

Telephone search—Assesses selective attention via ability to search for key symbols in a simulated classified telephone directory.

Telephone search dual task—Assesses divided attention via ability to search for key symbols in a simulated classified telephone directory while simultaneously counting strings of tape-presented tones.

continues

Table 5-1 continued

Test/Subtest	Process Assessed					
	Attention	Memory	Perception	Orientation	Higher Cognitive Processes	Communication: Pragmatics (PR)/ Semantics (S)
Lottery—Assesses sustained attention via ability to listen to a string of numbers and writing down the two letters preceding all numbers ending in "55." This test is normed on young and old normal subjects and patients with stroke, closed head injury, and Alzheimer's disease. Standardized scores allow comparisons across etiological groups in terms of selective, sustained, and alternating attention. The test has three parallel versions.	X					
Verbal and Nonverbal Cancellation Test, by M.M. Mesulam (1985). Available from: F.A. Davis, 404–420 N. 2nd Street, Philadelphia, PA 19123. Assesses directed attention via ability to identify a target in the following four test formats: the target *A* from letters arranged in rows and columns (structured verbal); the target *A* from letters randomly distributed across the page (unstructured verbal); the target "open circle with a slanted line through it" from geometric shapes arranged in rows and columns (structured nonverbal); and the target "open circle with a slanted line through it" from geometric shapes randomly distributed across the page (unstructured nonverbal).	X					

Guidelines for rate and accuracy of performance for normal adults (up to age 50 years, 50 to 80 years, and over 80 years) and individuals with right and left hemisphere lesions are available (Weintraub S, Mesulam MM. Mental state assessment of young and elderly adults in behavioral neurology. In: Mesulam MM, ed. *Principles of Behavioral Neurology*, Philadelphia, Pa: FA Davis; 1985: 71–123).

Visual Object and Space Perception Battery, by E. Warrington and M. James (1991), Thames Valley Test Company. Available from: Northern Speech Services, Inc., 117 North Elm Street, PO Box 1247, Gaylord, MI 49735.

Consists of an initial screening measure to ensure adequate visual shape discrimination and eight subtests each designed to assess a particular aspect of object or space perception.

Test 1: Incomplete Letters—Assesses ability to identify incomplete letter stimuli.

Test 2: Silhouettes—Assesses ability to recognize silhouettes of objects.

Test 3: Object Decision—Assesses ability to select a real object from distractors (nonobject designs).

Test 4: Progressive Silhouettes—Assesses ability to recognize an object from a series of silhouettes of the same object presented from a number of different angles.

Test 5: Dot Counting—Assesses ability to localize a single point and scan an array of black dots.

Test 6: Position Discrimination—Assesses ability to perceive the relative position of dots in two-dimensional space.

continues

Table 5-1 continued

Test/Subtest	Attention	Memory	Perception	Orientation	Higher Cognitive Processes	Communication: Pragmatics (PR)/ Semantics (S)
Test 7: Number Location—Assesses ability to identify the position of a dot in a square and match its position to one of nine numbers in another square.			X			
Test 8: Cube Analysis—Assesses complex spatial relationships in a three-dimensional arrangement of bricks.			X			
The test is standardized and validated on a group of normal controls and patients with right and left cerebral lesions. Normative data are available for ages 20 to 69.						
Woodcock-Johnson Psychoeducational Battery Revised by R.W. Woodcock and M.B. Johnson (1989). Available from: The Riverside Publishing Company, 8420 Bryn Mawr Avenue, Chicago, IL 60631.						
Test 1: Memory for Names—Assesses ability to learn associations between unfamiliar auditory and visual stimuli.		X				
Test 2: Memory for Sentences—Assesses ability to repeat phrases and sentences presented auditorily via a tape recorder.	X	X				
Test 5: Visual Closure—Assesses ability to identify a drawing or picture that is distorted, has missing lines or areas, or has a superimposed pattern.			X			

Test 9: Memory for Words—Assesses ability to repeat in correct sequence lists of unrelated words presented via a tape recorder.

Test 10: Cross Out—Assesses ability to scan and match visual information quickly.

Test 14: Concept Formation—Assesses ability to identify the rules for concepts when shown illustrations of when the rule does or does not apply.

Test 17: Numbers Reversed—Assesses ability to say in reverse order a series of numbers presented via a tape recorder.

Test 19: Spatial Relations—Assesses ability to identify from a series of shapes, the component parts of a given shape.

Test 20: Verbal Analogies—Assesses ability to complete phrases with words that indicate appropriate analogies.

The test is normed on more than 6,300 subjects ages 2 to 90+ years. Age-equivalent scores are available from ages 2 to 90+ and grade-equivalent scores are available from kindergarten through 16.9.

Chapter 6

Treatment of Cognitive-Communicative Skills in Patients with Right Hemisphere Damage

Anita S. Halper, Leora Reiff Cherney, and Martha S. Burns

INTRODUCTION

This chapter presents guidelines for treating the patient with right hemisphere damage and is organized by the cognitive processes discussed in Chapter 3. Within each process, long-term clinical objectives, short-term clinical objectives, procedures to achieve the short-term objectives, and a variety of measures of performance on the procedure are provided. Although the clinician is treating communication problems that are associated with problems in cognition, both long- and short-term objectives are written using terminology consistent with improving communication. For example, an attention objective written in cognitive terminology is "consistent ability to sustain attention to all activities during a 30-minute session." This may be rewritten as a communication goal of "consistent ability to attend to a 30-minute conversation." In addition, long-term objectives are functionally based, while short-term clinical objectives address the activities designed to achieve these functional outcomes. This emphasis on writing functional goals for communication is consistent with current trends and preferences of third-party payers.

There are certain treatment issues peculiar to this population that must be considered to ensure a positive therapeutic outcome. Prior to enrollment, the clinician must determine the patient's readiness and willingness to engage in an organized treatment program. This is particularly important given today's health care climate and limited number of treatment sessions typically authorized by third-party payers.

In order to participate in treatment, the patient must demonstrate a means of responding to stimuli. This response does not necessarily have to be appropriate, accurate, or consistent. The patient's medical condition will also affect the patient's readiness to engage in treatment. The patient's willingness to participate is associated with the ability to recognize deficits. Persistent unawareness and denial of deficits may negate a patient's continuing in a structured treatment program. The patient's denial of deficits can be controlled somewhat by careful organization of treatment goals and task levels. In addition, it is essential that the clinician be careful about establishing clear goals with the patient and family. Further, the clinician should objectively measure change in a way that the patient can see and understand. In some cases, the benefits to be gained from treatment will not outweigh the patient's frustration and desire to terminate therapy.

There is not a great deal of information available to the general public about the nature and extent of the cognitive-communicative problems in patients with right hemisphere damage. It is essential that the patient's family be instructed about the nature of the patient's limitations and types of deficits that may occur with this population. These include denial and lack of recognition of deficits, impulsivity, place and time disorientation, and problems with judgment and reasoning. Many patients will also exhibit lack of affect, which may result in an apparent disinterest in personal interactions. Deficits in visuospatial perception should be explained in terms of the effect on physical maneuvering, orientation, and reading and writing. Appendix 6–A provides guidelines for family and significant others for facilitating communication.

Family members and significant others are essential members of the treatment team. Goals should be mutually developed by the patient, family, and clinician. The patient's premorbid educational level, skills, interests, and discharge placement should be considered when setting therapeutic goals and developing procedures. Incorporation of the family into the therapeutic process at all stages will also help the family and patient adjust to the illness and maximize carryover.

When the clinician, patient, and family determine the long-term functional objectives, consideration of types of communication activities within the patient's own living or work environment is of prime importance. Living environments may include the following: home with round-the-clock supervision, home with supervision part of the day, home with minimal supervision, home alone, transitional living facility, and skilled nursing facility. Obviously the skills targeted for a patient at home and living alone will be different from someone in a skilled nursing facility. Similarly the skills targeted for patients with vocational goals will differ from the skills targeted for those who will not be employed. Vocational outcome may include the following: full- or part-time employment with no adjustment in hours or tasks, full- or part-time employment with adjusted hours and tasks, sheltered workshop, student, volunteer, homemaker, retired, and unemployed.

The organization of this chapter is a purely superficial one. Processes should not be thought of as clear-cut divisions, but rather as processing capabilities that must be considered for each task.

Therefore, clinicians may simultaneously address several cognitive processes that underlie the patient's communication failures. Not only does the surface communicative behavior improve but, presumably, the underlying cognitive processes are enhanced as well.

Accordingly, the goals and treatment procedures presented are meant as a guide, not an exhaustive list, for treatment of patients with cognitive-communicative deficits associated with right hemisphere damage. Some goals and procedures may be appropriate for patients in specific settings only (e.g., acute hospital, subacute unit, acute rehabilitation, home health, extended care facilities, outpatient, or day programs). Other goals and procedures may be appropriate for more than one setting. For example, in a subacute unit, clinicians may emphasize specific activities to improve focused and sustained attention to the environment. On the other hand, in an outpatient setting, attention may not be worked on directly but rather subsumed within other communication activities.

In addition to individual treatment, group treatment is an effective means of achieving the goals presented. This is particularly true for memory, orientation, and pragmatics. There are a variety of published materials and computer programs that can be used in both individual and group treatment for this population. Appendix 6–B lists the names, addresses, and telephone numbers of the major publishers of these materials. Specific lists of materials are not included because of the rapid changes in their availability.

ATTENTION

Attention is typically not singled out as a separate goal in the treatment of right hemisphere dysfunction because the attentional mechanisms affected by right hemisphere lesions are part of a processing circuit that affects attention, memory, communication, and reasoning components of cognition.[1] However, in certain settings, such as subacute rehabilitation, it may be appropriate to implement procedures that directly target attention skills.

The goals of treatment are to provide the patients with strategies to use independently in their functional environment. When attention is targeted directly, it should be done within the context of a functional activity. In addition, an important component is to instruct significant others about how to control for attentional problems within the patient's living environment or how to assist the patient in using strategies.

Attentional problems that may contribute to communication failure after right hemisphere lesions include difficulties with sustained attention, selective attention, division of attention between tasks, or attention to or exploration of the left side of space. The following goals represent illustrative examples of the ways attention can be addressed and documented within broader functional outcome objectives.

LONG-TERM CLINICAL OBJECTIVE

Patient demonstrates consistent attention to _____ minute conversation with or in _____ (e.g., number of people, noisy versus quiet environment, home setting, work setting).

Short-Term Clinical Objective	Procedure	Measurement	Comments
Increase selective attention to auditory instructions of _____ length in _____ environment (e.g., treatment, dining room, reception area)	Provide a set of instructions (e.g., how to get from one therapy to another, physical therapy instructions for transferring) with distractions that the patient might encounter in his or her own environment • Have patient follow the instructions • Experiment with visual and associative cueing techniques or compensatory techniques (see Exhibit 6–1) to determine which techniques aid selective attention for the tasks • Gradually increase length	Number and type of cues or compensatory tactics	

LONG-TERM CLINICAL OBJECTIVE

Patient demonstrates consistent attention to the left side of space during _____ activity (e.g., reading comprehension, written expression, conversation) in a _____ environment (e.g., home setting, work environment).

Short-Term Clinical Objective	Procedure	Measurement	Comments
Increase selective attention to the left side of space for visual objects and words in the _____ environment	Move into a new environmental setting (e.g., new room, nearby store, or rearranged room) and place a specified object in an unusual position • Have the patient scan the environment naming all objects observed until able to attend to the target object • Cue to the left as necessary	Number of repetitions or cues required to find the object and/or Time taken to scan the environment for the object	
	Create a route (e.g., from one room to another) and identify landmarks or directional signs on the left side for the patient to attend to during repetition of the route • Have patient repeat the route • Cue as needed by identifying the landmarks for the patient	Number of landmarks or directional signs attended to correctly and/or Number of cues required and/or Time taken to repeat the route	
	Use Myers and Mackisack's[2] Edgeness Program (see Exhibit 6–2)	As specified in program	This is a seven-step treatment procedure using blocks and a segment board to help the patient establish boundaries of relevant space and explore within these boundaries[2]

continues

Short-Term Clinical Objective	Procedure	Measurement	Comments
Increase selective distribution of attention to the left side of space for _____ (e.g., word, sentence, page) level of written material	Use Myer and Mackisack's[2] Bookness Program (see Exhibit 6–3)	As specified in program	This technique, similar to "Edgeness," described above, uses a book instead of blocks and a segment board

	Use scanning and tracking exercises to increase attention to the left side of the page
	• Modify stimuli by
	  1. Decreasing size of targets and foils
	  2. Increasing length of words
	  3. Increasing similarity between target and foils
	• Use cues such as the following:
	  1. Red orienting lines on the left and right
	  2. Guides to focus on a single line such as a card or ruler
	  3. Tactile markers such as velcro placed vertically or horizontally
	  4. Verbal reminders to orient to the left and move eyes to the right
		Percentage correct and/or Length of time patient sustains attention to task	Treatment stimuli for scanning and tracking activities are available in a variety of workbooks and in Attention Process Training Programs (APT[3] and APT–II[4]). These programs also have activities for addressing auditory attention.
			
			See Exhibit 6–4 for functional activities for scanning and tracking

LONG-TERM CLINICAL OBJECTIVE

Patient demonstrates consistent _____ (e.g., selective, alternating, divided) attention to _____ (e.g., words, sentence, page) level of written material for _____ (e.g., safety, leisure, work) purposes.

Short-Term Clinical Objective	Procedure	Measurement	Comments
Increase selective attention for _____ level written material	Use the previously mentioned scanning and tracking exercises • Introduce competing stimuli (e.g., radio, open door) • Increase gradually the amount of distraction • Use verbal, gestural, or tactile cues	Percentage correct and/or Length of time attention sustained to task and/or Type and number of cues required to maintain attention to task	Whenever possible use functional materials for all of the scanning and tracking exercises (see Exhibit 6–4)
Increase alternating attention for _____ level written material	Use the previously mentioned scanning and tracking exercises • Have patient alternate between two different task requirements (see Exhibit 6–5) • Increase the number of different tasks the patient must alternate between • Increase gradually the number of shifts required in a designated period of time	Percentage correct and/or Number of shifts in a designated period of time and/or Length of time required to change attention sets	
Increase divided attention to _____ level of written material	Use the above scanning and tracking exercises and introduce another activity (e.g., conversation, talking on telephone) • Have patient complete original task while simultaneously performing a new task	Percentage correct and/or Length of time patient attends to both activities simultaneously	

Exhibit 6–1 Types of Cues and Compensatory Tactics

Associative and Visual Cues*

- Written instructions
- Simplified words
- Numbering of steps
- Pictured illustrations of steps
- Rhymes, rhythms, or musical cues
- Visual and tactile cues to the left
- Visual aids for route finding

Compensatory Attentional Tactics*

- Request repetition
- Repeat instruction aloud
- Use fingers to count or guide each step
- Create a motor image through practice
- Create a visual image of each step
- Cue verbally to the left
- Self create visual plans

*Many of these adaptations are used naturally and routinely by most clinicians during treatment. The above format simply permits including these as part of a goal statement and, thereby, accurately accounting for functional outcome gains.

Exhibit 6–2 Edgeness Program

PURPOSE

Assist patient in determining the boundaries of relevant space and performing tasks within that space

MATERIALS

- Flat board or grid divided into four, six, or eight equal segments
- Segments are marked by grooves that provide the patient with tactile cues to establish boundaries
- DLM 1 inch colored cubes

PROCEDURE

- Stage 1
  1. Patient traces edge of grid with fingers and follows tracing with eyes
  2. Patient looks away; clinician places single cube in center of top right segment
  3. Patient looks at grid, finds cube, and gives it to clinician
  4. Clinician places cube for patient to find in varying locations (top right, lower right, upper left, and lower left segments in that order); cube is moved systematically within the segment from center out and from top to bottom
- Stage 2
  1. Clinician places two cubes of the same color on either side of midline, one in the top right segment and the other in the top left segment
  2. Patient retrieves both cubes
- Stage 3
  1. Clinician places one cube next to midline in top left segment; the other cube is moved progressively farther out to the edge of the top right segment

continues

Exhibit 6–2 continued

    2. Patient retrieves both cubes each time the right cube is moved
    3. Repeat above steps in the lower segments
- Stage 4
Repeat Stage 3 with right cube placed close to midline and left cube being moved progressively out to the edge
- Stage 5
    1. Clinician randomly mixes order of placement of two cubes for patient to retrieve
    2. Gradually increase the number of pairs of colored cubes (to a maximum of eight) for patient to retrieve
- Stage 6
    1. Clinician places a random number (e.g., three, five) of the same-colored cubes on either side of midline; initially use only upper or lower segments for patient to retrieve
    2. Later, vary location
- Stage 7
    1. Clinician increases number of segments in grid to six or eight
    2. Repeat above stages

MEASUREMENT

- Three accurate retrievals out of four per placement before moving to the next stage
- In all stages, patient uses visual and tactile tracing of the edge of the grid before each retrieval; cues are gradually faded

Source: Reprinted with permission from P.S. Myers and E.L. Mackisack, "Right Hemisphere Syndrome," in *Aphasia and Related Neurogenic Language Disorders*, L.L. LaPointe, ed., pp. 177–195, © 1990, Thieme Medical Publishers, Inc.

Exhibit 6–3 Bookness Program

PURPOSE

Assist patient in recognizing the boundaries of a closed and open book

MATERIALS

Thick book

PROCEDURE

- Place thick, closed book at the patient's midline
- Have patient describe the physical characteristics of the book and explain how we read (left to right, top to bottom, use of margins)
- Have patient trace the edge of the book, following with the eyes and describing what is seen
- Repeat above steps with book open
- Have patient match a stimulus on the left page with one of four stimuli on the right page; initially use shapes and letters until patient can progress to words and sentences
- Increase number of foils and decrease space between stimuli

MEASUREMENT

- Not provided by authors
- Matching tasks can be measured by percentage correct
- Patient traces the edge of the book before each activity; cues are gradually faded

Source: Reprinted with permission from P.S. Myers and E.L. Mackisack, "Right Hemisphere Syndrome," in *Aphasia and Related Neurogenic Language Disorders*, L.L. LaPointe, ed., pp. 177–195, © 1990, Thieme Medical Publishers, Inc.

Exhibit 6–4 Functional Materials for Scanning and Tracking

- Bus, train, or airline schedules
- Catalogs
- Dictionary
- Directions on food packages
- Grocery lists
- Local magazine or newspaper listings of activities (e.g., movies, restaurants, museums)
- Maps
- Menus
- Newspaper ads
- Newspaper headlines
- Newspaper listings of national and foreign weather information
- Nutritional information on food products
- Phone book
- Racing form
- Recipes
- Table of contents
- TV guide
- Vending machines

Exhibit 6–5 Sample Tasks for Shifting Attention

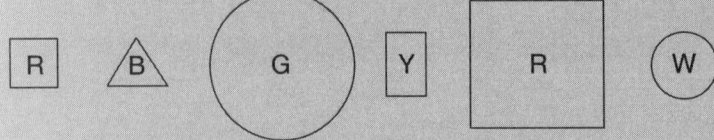

Task 1—Patient identifies a specific shape (e.g., all squares)

Task 2—Patient identifies a specific color (e.g., all red items)

Task 3—Patient identifies a specific size (e.g., all large items)

ALCqERFnNMRoSyzPmqLtdNZe

Task 1—Patient identifies all upper case letters

Task 2—Patient identifies all lower case letters

Task 3—Patient identifies all vowels

Task 4—Patient identifies all consonants

---

cat show red nice dog nine jacket yellow

Task 1—Patient identifies all items in a specific category (e.g., animals)

Task 2—Patient identifies all words that end in "e"

Task 3—Patient identifies all two-syllable words

PERCEPTION

Treatment in the area of perception should focus on perceptual skills necessary for communication including effective communication interaction, reading, writing, and calculation skills. Long-term functional objectives depend on the patient's vocational and avocational goals and the patient's interaction needs in the family and community. It should be noted that activities for the perception of the nonverbal aspects of communication discussed in this section are useful for treatment of pragmatics. In addition, the activities and cues for scanning and tracking and for increasing attention to the left side of space are also useful for treatment of perception.

LONG-TERM CLINICAL OBJECTIVE

Patient demonstrates consistent perception of nonverbal _____ (e.g., facial, prosodic, body) cues during a _____ minute conversation with _____ (number) people.

Short-Term Clinical Objective	Procedure	Measurement	Comments
Consistent perception of _____ (number) facial characteristics and expressions in _____ (e.g., photographs, cartoons, videotapes) for effective communicative interactions	Present the patient with a photograph, cartoon, or videotape • Have patient identify distinctive features (e.g., hair color, eye color, dimples, freckles, wrinkles, buckteeth) • Move from familiar to unfamiliar faces	Ratio of number of features identified to actual number of features	
	Present the patient with a photograph, cartoon, or videotape • Have patient identify expressions (e.g., angry, sad, happy, surprised) • Move from obvious to more subtle expressions	Percentage correct	
	Present the patient with a photograph, cartoon, or videotape; have patient listen to a sentence and determine whether the inflection matches the facial expression	Percentage correct	

continues

Short-Term Clinical Objective	Procedure	Measurement	Comments
Consistent perception of body posture in _____ (e.g., photographs, cartoons, videotapes) for effective communicative interactions	Present the patient with a photograph, cartoon, or videotape • Have patient identify the emotional intent (e.g., anger, fear, joy) of the body posture • Move from obvious to more subtle emotional intents	Percentage correct	
	Present the patient with a photograph, cartoon, or videotape • Have patient determine whether the body posture matches the facial expression • Have patient listen to a sentence and determine whether the inflection matches the body posture	Percentage correct Percentage correct	
Consistent perception of facial expression and body posture in situational contexts	Present the patient with a photograph, cartoon, or videotape of an individual in a scene; have patient identify whether the body posture and facial expression are appropriate for the scene and indicate why	Percentage correct	
Consistent perception of nonverbal facial expression, prosody, and body posture in conversation	Provide patient with instructions to respond to a specified nonverbal cue in a conversation (e.g., begin speaking when you hear my voice drop signaling the end of my turn); videotape the conversation and have the patient provide feedback about the appropriateness of the response	Percentage of appropriate responses	

LONG-TERM CLINICAL OBJECTIVE

Patient demonstrates consistent spatial organization for writing of _____ (e.g., words, sentences, paragraphs, numbers) in _____ (e.g., grocery list, letter, work-related report, checkbook).

Short-Term Clinical Objective	Procedure	Measurement	Comments
Consistent spatial organization of _____ (e.g., words, sentences) with _____ cues	Present patient with a guide for spacing words and sentences (see Figure 6–1); initially, the guide should have red or raised lines in horizontal or vertical positions • Have the patient copy words spaced correctly in the lines; progress to writing words to dictation and spontaneous writing of words (e.g., lists) • Gradually decrease line cues • Gradually increase length of patient's written response to phrases and sentences	Percentage of target items spaced correctly in the lines	
Consistent spatial organization of _____ (number) paragraphs with _____ cues	Have patient write a paragraph(s) (e.g., describing a picture, personal event) • Have patient identify the errors in spatial organization and provide cues as needed • Have patient rewrite sample and provide cues, as needed, to indicate the borders of the paragraph	Percentage correct Ratio of number of errors in corrected sample versus number in original sample	

continues

Short-Term Clinical Objective	Procedure	Measurement	Comments
Consistent spatial organization of columns in calculation tasks of _____ (e.g., addition, subtraction)	Have patient perform a calculation task; assist patient in maintaining columns using red or raised lines in combination with the following: • Lines and boxes (see Figure 6–2) • Graph paper • Lined paper Decrease gradually use of line cues Present the patient with a checkbook register • Have patient write items in the appropriate columns (e.g., check number, payment amount, balance) from a verbal or written stimulus • Have patient perform hypothetical checkbook transactions	Percentage of target items spaced correctly Percentage correct Percentage of items correctly spaced in columns	

Treatment of Cognitive-Communicative Skills 71

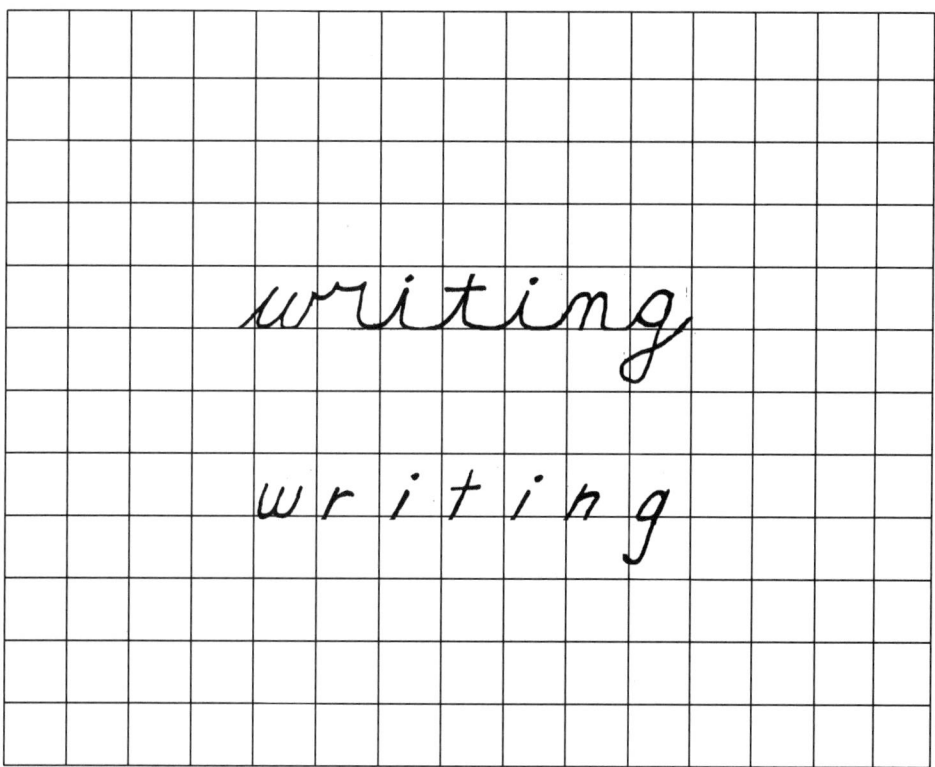

Figure 6–1 Spatial guide for writing

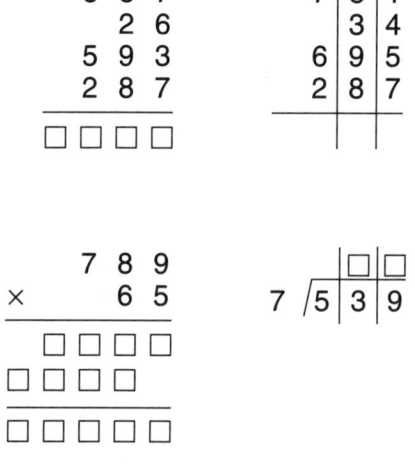

Figure 6–2 Spatial guide for maintaining columns for calculation

MEMORY

Memory problems can occur in any one or more of the processes of encoding, storage, or retrieval. Treatment strategies can be tailored to the area where the level of breakdown occurs. We believe that in the right hemisphere breakdown occurs primarily at the level of encoding.[5] Therefore, treatment techniques that will facilitate improvement in encoding are discussed.

Memory rehabilitation has been divided into two approaches: (1) restoration, and (2) compensation. Restoration focuses on improving memory through the use of exercises and drills. In contrast, compensation teaches the use of strategies to compensate for the memory loss. In terms of functional memory, only minimal improvements are evident following the use of a restoration approach.[6]

According to Sohlberg and Mateer,[6] there are two types of compensatory strategies: (1) external compensatory strategies (e.g., calendar, clock, memory book), and (2) internal compensatory strategies (e.g., mnemonics, chunking). Treatment should stress the use of external strategies and the generalization of their use to the natural environment. Internal compensatory strategies are useful for facilitating the retention of small amounts of specific information that is important to the patient. The clinician should not expect the patient to spontaneously use internal strategies functionally to recall large amounts of general information.

Treatment for memory will only be successful if the patient is aware of the memory problems and is motivated to use the compensatory strategies. Therefore, one of the first goals of treatment is to facilitate increased awareness of the problem. However, there are different degrees of awareness and it is important to select a compensatory strategy that matches the patient's level of awareness (see Exhibit 6–6). Exhibit 6–7 provides a list of functional stimuli that can be used for many of the following treatment procedures.

Exhibit 6–6 Types of Awareness and Related Compensation Techniques

AWARENESS	DEFINITION
Intellectual	Ability to understand at some level that a particular function is impaired
Emergent	Ability to recognize a problem only when it is actually occurring
Anticipatory	Ability to anticipate that a problem will occur in a particular situation as a result of a particular deficit

COMPENSATION	DEFINITION
External	Strategies initiated by someone other than the patient or that may involve modifying the environment; does not require any of the above levels of awareness
Situational	Strategies that are triggered by specific situations or events in which deficits are likely to occur; requires intellectual awareness
Recognition	Strategies that are triggered by the patient's recognition that a problem is occurring; requires emergent awareness
Anticipatory	Strategies that are triggered by the patient's anticipation that a problem will occur if the strategy is not used; requires anticipatory awareness

Source: Reprinted with permission from B. Crosson, P.P. Barco, C.A. Velzo et al., Awareness and Compensation in Postacute Head Injury Rehabilitation, *Journal of Head Trauma Rehabilitation*, Volume 4, No. 3, pp. 46–54, © 1989, Aspen Publishers, Inc.

Exhibit 6–7 Functional Stimuli for Memory Procedures

NEW INFORMATION

- Headline of a current event
- Someone's address
- Names of new acquaintances
- Title and performers of new movies, TV shows, and plays
- Title and author of new books
- New schedule
  1. TV program
  2. Train, bus, or airplane schedule
  3. Treatment schedule
- Today's weather
- Current traffic report
- Phone message
- Instructions for
  1. Taking medications
  2. Operating a new appliance (e.g., microwave oven, VCR, cellular phone, voice mail)
  3. Getting to a specific location
  4. A new recipe
- Names and scores of winning teams (e.g., baseball, basketball, football)
- Daily lotto or lottery numbers
- Balance of checking or savings accounts

TYPES OF LISTS

- Items to purchase at specific stores (e.g., grocery store, department store, hardware store, drug store)
- Errands to run
- Categories of food (e.g., types of fruits, vegetables, meats, and bakery goods)
- Names of significant others (e.g., grandchildren, children)
- Current movies playing
- Clothes to take to the cleaners
- Items to pack for a trip
- Things to do at work or at home
- Things for a service person to do in your home (e.g., TV repairman, lawn service, babysitter)
- Questions to ask a professional person (e.g., your doctor, your accountant, your lawyer)

LONG-TERM CLINICAL OBJECTIVE

Patient demonstrates consistent comprehension and expression of _____ (type of information—e.g., daily activities, current events) in a _____ minute conversation using compensatory strategy(ies) of _____ (type—e.g., memory book, mnemonic).

Short-Term Clinical Objective	Procedure	Measurement	Comments
Increase awareness of the memory problem and need to use compensatory strategies for comprehension and expression of a simple piece of information after _____ minutes	Provide the patient with a simple piece of information • Instruct the patient to recall the information after a designated period of time during which you know the patient would have forgotten the information • Stress to the patient that although this information has been forgotten, there are compensatory strategies that can be used to help remember certain information	Ratio of the number of times patient was aware information was forgotten to the number of times the information was actually forgotten	This activity may need to be repeated several times during the session and over a period of time, varying the information to be remembered
Increase awareness of the memory problem and need to use compensatory strategies for comprehension of a daily activity or simple task after _____ minutes	Present a simple task (see Exhibit 6–8) • Instruct the patient to perform the task after a designated period of time in which you know the patient would have forgotten the task • Stress to the patient that although the task was not completed, there are compensatory strategies that can be used to help remember to perform the task	Ratio of the number of times patient was aware that the task was not completed to the number of times the task was actually forgotten	This activity may need to be repeated several times during the session and over a period of time, varying the tasks to be completed

continues

Short-Term Clinical Objective	Procedure	Measurement	Comments
Increase awareness of the memory problem and need to use compensatory strategies for expression of the location of an item after _____ minutes	Hide a personal item of the patient (e.g., handkerchief, pen) while patient watches where it is hidden • Instruct the patient to find the item after a designated period of time during which you know the patient would have forgotten the location • Stress to the patient that although the information has been forgotten there are compensatory strategies that can be used to help remember certain information	Ratio of the number of times patient was aware of failure to remember the location of the item to the number of times the location was forgotten	This procedure and the preceding one are appropriate for group treatment
Provide strategies to facilitate comprehension and expression of new information after _____ minutes	Provide the patient with a new piece of information (e.g., headline of a current event, an address, new schedule) • Have patient rehearse orally for a designated period of time, gradually decrease the length of time of rehearsal • Have patient provide the information on request • Gradually increase the length of time between giving the information or completing the rehearsal and requesting the information	Length of time required for rehearsal and Length of time patient is able to retain information	This task, and all of the following tasks, provide opportunities to teach the patients strategies that will facilitate encoding. These tasks are not arranged in a hierarchical fashion. Not all of the strategies will be useful to a particular patient. The clinician should explore those strategies that best facilitate encoding for a given patient.

continues

Short-Term Clinical Objective	Procedure	Measurement	Comments
	Provide the patient with a new piece of information and have patient write it down in an external compensatory device (e.g., calendar, memory book, diary) • Have patient provide the information on request • Gradually increase the length of time between writing it down and requesting the information	Percentage correct of information recalled and Type and number of cues required to retrieve information	
	Present a piece of information (e.g., today's weather including temperature; traffic report) and help the patient to analyze the information by attaching deep meaning to it (e.g., need sunglasses, coat, umbrella, boots, or hat; changing departure time or changing route) • Have patient provide the information on request • Gradually increase the length of time between giving the information or completing the rehearsal and requesting the information • Progress from clinician- to patient-generated analyses of meaning	Length of time patient is able to retain information and/or Number of self-generated versus clinician-generated analyses	This memory strategy of deep analysis requires the patient to use reasoning skills

continues

Short-Term Clinical Objective	Procedure	Measurement	Comments
	Present a list (e.g., grocery items; errands) or telephone number and have the patient group the items in order to reduce the number of informational units to be remembered (e.g., group associated items together, such as dairy products, baked goods, cleaners; chunk telephone numbers into two or three units) • Have patient provide the information on request • Gradually increase the length of time between giving the information and requesting the information • Progress from clinician- to patient-generated grouping strategies	Length of time patient is able to retain information and/or Number of self-generated versus clinician-generated grouping strategies	
	Present a list (e.g., grocery items in the same category such as fruit, grandchildren's names) and organize the items (e.g., alphabetically, by size or age) • Have patient provide the information on request • Gradually increase the length of time between giving the information and requesting the information • Progress from clinician- to patient-generated organizing strategies	Length of time patient is able to retain information and/or Number of self-generated versus clinician-generated organizing strategies	
	Present a new piece of auditory or visual information • Direct the patient to listen or look for specific information prior to or after presentation of the information • Gradually increase the length of the information presented • Gradually decrease the number of directed listening or reading cues	Percentage correct of pertinent information recalled and number of cues required	

Exhibit 6–8 Tasks To Be Performed After a Designated Period of Time

- Watering the plants
- Opening the door
- Making a phone call
- Finding a specific item in the room
- Putting a book back on the book shelf
- Writing own name and address on the piece of paper on the desk
- Making an entry on the desk calendar
- Finding a specific person's phone number in the hospital phone directory
- Putting a message in a specific mailbox in the office
- Getting a cup of coffee

ORIENTATION

Orientation is not a basic cognitive process but rather results from the integration of attention, memory, and perception as well as the higher cognitive processes. Regardless of the cause of the orientation deficit, the use of compensatory techniques may effectively reduce the impact of the disorder in day-to-day functional situations. In addition, treatment may focus on the underlying impaired processes that contribute to the problems in orientation. Compensatory procedures are discussed in this section; process-specific approaches are addressed under the appropriate process.

External compensatory strategies are useful for the treatment of orientation. Sohlberg and Mateer[6] have organized external compensatory strategies into three types: (1) multicomponent organizational aids, which assist an individual in organizing, storing, and retrieving relatively large amounts of information; (2) simple prospective devices, which remind a person to perform an activity at a specific time in the future; and (3) environmental modifications, which reduce the effect of the memory problems on day-to-day functional activities. A similar framework can be used to categorize external compensatory strategies for treatment of orientation. Rather than simple prospective devices, we prefer to call this category simple orientation aids because they serve as a method to facilitate the patient's orientation to time, place, and person.

Multicomponent organization devices include electronic notebook systems and computers. Simple orientation devices include such things as calendars, clock, watches, alarms, and floor plans. Environmental modifications might include such strategies as labeled shelves, post-it notes on a mirror, and alphabetized cabinets.

When selecting an external compensatory strategy, the clinician needs to consider the preferences of the individual, the family, and others in the environment. In addition, the specific cognitive and physical deficits of the patient will affect the type of strategy selected. Cognitive deficits include such deficits as reduced attention, slow information processing, reduced language comprehension, reduced problem-solving skills, and problems with executive functions. Physical deficits might include upper-extremity involvement and visual deficits.[7]

Burns, Halper, and Mogil[8] previously addressed treatment strategies for active orientation to time and place in the section on orientation. Since these skills also involve higher-level cognitive processes including organization and planning, treatment for these will be discussed in the section under that heading.

LONG-TERM CLINICAL OBJECTIVE

Patient demonstrates consistent ability to comprehend and express _____ (e.g., time, place, person) orientation information using an external compensatory strategy or environmental cues in a _____ (e.g., home, work) environment.

Short-Term Clinical Objective	Procedure	Measurement	Comments
Consistent comprehension and expression of the purpose and component parts of an external orientation (time, place, and person) compensatory strategy	Review the purpose of the orientation device and demonstrate its component parts; ask questions regarding the device using a variety of question–answer formats (e.g., yes or no, multiple choice, open-ended)	Percentage of correct responses to questions regarding the external device	

continues

Short-Term Clinical Objective	Procedure	Measurement	Comments
Consistent expression of _____ (e.g., time, place, person) orientation information using an external compensatory strategy in a clinical setting	Provide the patient with situations (e.g., making an appointment, taking medication at a specific time, meeting a new acquaintance) in which expression of orientation information is required; have the patient use the external compensatory strategy to express or demonstrate the orientation information	Percentage of correct responses expressing orientation information using an external compensatory device	Rather than asking the patient questions, such as what is the date, time, or place, it is preferable to present functional situations pertinent to the patient to elicit this information. For example, present two newspapers and have the patient select today's paper; or select a TV program based on date and time.
Consistent expression of _____ (e.g., time, place, person) orientation information using an external compensatory strategy in a role-playing situation	Provide the patient with situations (e.g., making an appointment, meeting a new acquaintance) in which expression of orientation information is required; have the patient role-play the situation using the external compensatory strategy to express the orientation information	Percentage of correct responses expressing orientation information using an external compensatory device	This procedure is appropriate for group treatment
Consistent expression of _____ (e.g., time, place, person) orientation information using an external compensatory strategy in a natural setting	Put the patient in situations (e.g., nursing unit, cafeteria, grocery store) in which expression of orientation information is required; have the patient use the external compensatory strategy to express the orientation information	Percentage of correct responses expressing orientation information using an external compensatory device	

continues

Short-Term Clinical Objective	Procedure	Measurement	Comments
Consistent ability to express _____ (e.g., time and place) orientation information using environmental cues	Present environmental cues for time (e.g., dark versus light, snow versus green grass) and for place (e.g., white coats and stethoscope to indicate hospital, stove and refrigerator to indicate kitchen) • Have patient answer questions regarding the above • Move from maximal cueing by the clinician to patient self-generated cues	Percentage of correct responses to questions and/or Type and number of clinician-generated cues and/or Number of self-generated versus clinician-generated cues	

PRAGMATICS

Impairments in pragmatics of communication are viewed as a major characteristic of the cognitive–communicative deficits resulting from right hemisphere damage.[9] Disturbances may occur in any of three contexts: (1) extralinguistic, (2) paralinguistic, and (3) linguistic, as described in Chapter 3. Extralinguistic problems occur in nonverbal behaviors such as gestures, body posture, eye contact, and facial expression. The paralinguistic problems are reflected in intonation and prosody. Linguistic deficits occur in the patient's discourse, such as conversation and storytelling. With some patients, the clinician will focus on each pragmatic area separately, whereas with others the treatment can be integrated to include more than one of the above contexts. It is important for the clinician to note that many of the procedures for direct intervention of pragmatics may be appropriate for only a select group of patients, particularly those considering returning to a work or school environment.

Rather, the clinician should consider pragmatic communication deficits when treating all of the processes. For example, when the focus of treatment is establishing attention, working on such tasks as attending to a speaker or shifting attention from one speaker to another will impact on pragmatic skills as well as attention. Such tasks facilitate improved eye contact in conversation. Similarly, when the focus of treatment is to improve memory, such tasks as learning compensatory strategies for retaining information will facilitate improved topic maintenance.

This section presents procedures for the direct treatment of the linguistic context of pragmatics. These procedures are consistent with the three-phase training model for pragmatics: (1) awareness, (2) practice, and (3) generalization, described by Sohlberg and her colleagues.[10] Treatment of the paralinguistic and the extralinguistic contexts are included in the sections on attention and perception. When a patient requires cues to achieve a short-term goal, the cueing should be included in the goal. In addition, the type and number of cues required in a designated period of time is an appropriate measure of patient performance.

The treatment of pragmatic problems often can be more effective in group situations where more natural interactions can occur. Practicing pragmatic skills in a group setting can facilitate generalization. Group interactions can be captured on videotapes and replayed for the group members to analyze. Videotaping and using scripts can be incorporated into a number of the procedures described below. Involving families and other caregivers in the treatment process and training them as effective communication partners is also necessary to facilitate generalization to natural settings (see Exhibit 6–9).

Exhibit 6–9 Training Families and Caregivers As Effective Communication Partners

- Ask the patient pertinent background information about the topic being discussed; supply the same kind of information when the patient is in the listener role
- Ask the patient to explain the relevance of a contribution, and provide explicit linkages to the present topic for the patient
- Restate, ask questions to reestablish, or otherwise cue the topic under discussion
- Provide focused and consistent requests for clarification, specifying the trouble source for the patient
- Prompt or signal the patient to focus on main ideas and central information
- Emphasize essential information using the modalities (e.g., gestures, writing) and utterance forms that the patient can interpret most readily
- Use or prompt the patient to use turn-taking, topic-shifting, or conversation-closing signals that are overt, clear, and explicit
- Remind the patient to check whether a listener has understood
- Reduce rate and complexity of questions asked or information provided

Source: Reprinted with permission from C.A. Tompkins, *Right Hemisphere Communication Disorders: Theory and Management*, p. 278, © 1995, Singular Publishing Group, Inc.

LONG-TERM CLINICAL OBJECTIVE

Patient demonstrates consistent comprehension and expression of information in a _____ minute _____ (discourse type, e.g., conversation, storytelling, procedural tasks) using appropriate _____ (e.g., turn taking, topic maintenance).

Short-Term Clinical Objective	Procedure	Measurement	Comments
Increase awareness of disturbances in turn taking and need to make modifications in a _____ minute conversation	Review cues for turn taking (see Exhibit 6–10); have patient answer questions regarding use of cues	Percentage correct	
	Present a script of a conversation • Have the patient identify correct and incorrect instances of turn taking and explain why • Increase gradually the number of speakers in the script	Percentage correct	

continues

Short-Term Clinical Objective	Procedure	Measurement	Comments
	Present a videotape of a conversation between two people • Have the patient identify correct and incorrect instances of turn taking and explain why • Increase gradually the number of speakers in the script	Percentage correct	
	Present a videotape of a conversation between the patient and another individual • Have the patient identify correct and incorrect instances of turn taking and explain why • Increase gradually the number of speakers in the script	Percentage correct	
Increase awareness of disturbances in topic maintenance and need to make modifications in a _____ minute conversation	Present a topic and two statements • Have the patient identify whether each statement matches the topic • Increase gradually the number of statements presented	Percentage correct	
	Present a script of a conversation • Have patient identify the main topic(s) of the conversation • Have the patient identify instances of topic maintenance and topic change • Have patient identify whether these topic changes were smooth or abrupt	Percentage correct	

continues

Short-Term Clinical Objective	Procedure	Measurement	Comments
	Present a videotape of a conversation • Have patient identify the main topic(s) of the conversation • Have patient identify instances of topic maintenance and topic change • Have patient identify whether these topic changes were smooth or abrupt	Percentage correct	
Consistent comprehension and expression of information in a _____ minute conversation using appropriate turn-taking skills in a _____ (e.g., clinical, functional) setting	Have a conversation with the patient and videotape • Use cues (e.g., card with green and red dot, holding up your hand to stop) to signal to the patient when to take a turn and when to relinquish a turn • Gradually decrease the number of cues and modify the type of cues making them more subtle (e.g., eye contact or body posture rather than the more overt cues described above)	Number of appropriate and inappropriate turn-taking maneuvers in a designated period of time and/or Type and number of cues required in a designated time period	
	Have a conversation with the patient and videotape • Have patient and clinician evaluate patient's turn-taking skills at the end of the conversation • Have patient view the videotape to verify self-evaluation of turn-taking skills	Number of appropriate and inappropriate turn-taking maneuvers in a designated period of time and/or Percentage of agreement between the clinician's and patient's evaluation of turn-taking skills	

continues

Short-Term Clinical Objective	Procedure	Measurement	Comments
Consistent comprehension and expression of information in a _____ minute conversation in a natural setting using appropriate turn-taking skills	Put the patient in functional situations (e.g., cafeteria, making a telephone call) in which conversations are required; have the patient use turn-taking skills appropriately and self-monitor	Number of appropriate and inappropriate turn-taking maneuvers in a designated period of time and/or Percentage of agreement between the clinician's and patient's evaluation of turn-taking skills	
Consistent comprehension and expression of information in a _____ minute conversation using appropriate topic maintenance skills in a _____ (e.g., clinical, functional) setting	Have a conversation with the patient and videotape • Have patient and clinician evaluate patient's topic-maintenance skills at the end of the conversation • Have patient view the videotape to verify self-evaluation of own topic maintenance skills and explain how specific comments relate to the topic under discussion • Have patient practice correcting the nonmeaningful comments	Number of times patient appropriately initiated, maintained, or shifted topic in a designated period of time and/or Percentage of agreement between the clinician's and patient's evaluation of topic-maintenance skills	Topic-maintenance skills can be evaluated according to the following: • Function of the statement—initiation, maintenance, and shift • Informational content—meaningful versus nonmeaningful (irrelevant, off-topic, incorrect)

continues

Short-Term Clinical Objective	Procedure	Measurement	Comments
	Put the patient in functional situations (e.g., cafeteria, making a telephone call) in which conversations are required; have the patient maintain topic appropriately, self-monitor, and correct the nonmeaningful comments	Number of times patient appropriately initiated, maintained, or shifted topic in a designated period of time and/or Percentage of agreement between the clinician's and patient's evaluation of topic-maintenance skills	
Consistent expression of information in a _____ minute retelling of a personal experience	Present a script of a story • Have the patient identify the main idea of the story versus the details • Cue by providing a skeleton outline for the patient to complete • Have the patient identify meaningful and nonmeaningful information	Percentage correct	
	Present the patient with any of the following stimuli: picture card series; picture scene (e.g., Norman Rockwell picture); story that is heard or read; or a personal experience • Have the patient provide the main idea and details of the story • Use cues that facilitate expression of the general setting of the story, the major actions of the story, and the consequences or resolution of these actions	Ratio of the number of appropriate responses to inappropriate responses	

continues

Short-Term Clinical Objective	Procedure	Measurement	Comments
	Have the patient tell a story from any of the following stimuli: picture card series; picture scene (e.g., Norman Rockwell picture); story that is heard or read; or a personal experience	Amount of meaningful and nonmeaningful information produced in a designated period of time and/or Ratio of amount of meaningful information produced to total number of words	This task can be used in a group setting; each patient takes a turn and adds to the story
Appropriate expression of pronouns in a _____ minute _____ (conversation or retelling of a personal experience)	Present a picture that consists of two people • Have the patient identify each person by name or gender (e.g., man, woman) • Have the patient tell what each person is doing using appropriate pronouns • Modify the stimuli by increasing the number of individuals in the picture • Cue by asking questions about what the individuals in the picture are doing	Percentage correct of appropriate pronouns produced	Self-monitoring and self-evaluation should be incorporated into these treatment procedures
	Have the patient retell a personal experience; cue by asking questions about who the participants in the story are and what they are doing	Percentage correct of appropriate pronouns produced	
	Set up a barrier task and have the patient provide directions to the clinician or other patients in a group setting; cue by asking questions when instructions are unclear	Percentage correct of appropriate pronouns produced	Barrier tasks could include giving directions to draw or manipulate objects; the receiver of the information has no prior knowledge of the task to be completed

continues

Short-Term Clinical Objective	Procedure	Measurement	Comments
Appropriate expression of conjunctions in a ____ minute ____ (conversation or retelling of a personal experience)	Present the patient with a script that contains brief sentences • Have the patient use appropriate conjunctions to connect pairs of sentences • Gradually increase the length of the script	Percentage correct of appropriate conjunctions produced	Self-monitoring and self-evaluation should be incorporated into these treatment procedures
	Set up a barrier task and have the patient provide directions to the clinician or other patients in a group setting; cue by asking questions when instructions are unclear	Percentage correct of appropriate conjunctions produced	

Exhibit 6–10 Turn-Taking Cues

TURN-TAKING CUES THAT SIGNAL A DESIRE TO SPEAK

- Taking a deep breath
- Producing a transitional comment
- Initiating a gesture
- Shifting eye gaze away from the speaker
- Speaking simultaneously

TURN-TAKING CUES THAT SIGNAL A DESIRE TO RELINQUISH A TURN

- Pausing
- Reducing pitch
- Reducing loudness
- Completing a hand gesture
- Establishing eye contact with a listener

Source: Reprinted with permission from C.A. Tompkins, *Right Hemisphere Communication Disorders: Theory and Management*, p. 278, © 1995, Singular Publishing Group, Inc.

HIGHER-LEVEL COGNITIVE PROCESSES (ORGANIZATION, REASONING, AND PROBLEM SOLVING OR JUDGMENT)

There are several factors that should be considered when developing goals and procedures for organization, reasoning, and problem solving or judgment. These include the patient's educational and vocational level, and premorbid interests and cognitive abilities. In addition, higher-level cognitive skills may not be critical for functional adaptation in the environment. Rather, individuals who aspire to educational or vocational reentry may require these skills for performance effectiveness in the employment or academic arena. Furthermore, many of the tasks presented may be appropriate only for the mildly impaired patient with demonstrated potential for improvement in higher cognitive abilities.

LONG-TERM CLINICAL OBJECTIVE

Patient demonstrates consistent organization of written information for _____ (e.g., letters, note taking, and written narratives) for _____ (e.g., educational, vocational, avocational) purposes.

Short-Term Clinical Objective	Procedure	Measurement	Comments
Consistent organization of _____ (number) words into a sequential order	Present patient with a set of words • Have patient arrange the words in the correct order based on specified criteria (e.g., time—morning, evening, afternoon; size—foot, inch, yard; alphabetizing) • Cue by questioning the rationale for sequencing the items	Percentage correct and/or Accuracy of rationale for sequencing	
Consistent organization of _____ (number) _____ (sentences, paragraphs) into a meaningful narrative	Present several related sentences (e.g., steps for carrying out an activity, story) out of order • Have patient reorder the sentences into a meaningful sequence • Increase gradually the number of sentences presented	Percentage correct	

continues

Short-Term Clinical Objective	Procedure	Measurement	Comments
	Present several related paragraphs out of order • Have patient reorder the paragraphs into a meaningful narrative • Increase gradually the number of paragraphs presented	Percentage correct	
Consistent production of a _____ (number) component outline from a _____ (auditorily, visually) presented _____ (e.g., lecture, news article, newscast)	Present material (e.g., article, newscast, lecture) visually or auditorily • Have the patient identify the main idea, subtopics, details • Cue with questions or provide a partially completed or blank outline for the specific information given (see Exhibit 6–11) • Increase gradually the length of the material presented • Increase gradually the number of main ideas, subtopics, and details	Percentage correct or Number and type of cues required	
Consistent note taking of _____ (number) key elements of a _____ (auditorily, visually) presented _____ (e.g., lecture, newscast, physician instructions)	Present information auditorily or visually; have patient take notes enumerating the salient points	Percentage of salient facts included and/or Percentage correctly ordered	
Consistent prioritization of _____ (number) components of an activity according to a specified set of criteria	Present a situation (e.g., running errands, getting ready in the morning) (See Exhibit 6–12); have patient prioritize items according to specific salient features (e.g., cost, geographic location)	Number of details included and/or Percentage of agreement between the clinician and the patient	

continues

Short-Term Clinical Objective	Procedure	Measurement	Comments
Consistent expression of the sequence of steps and time required for the completion of a functional daily activity	Present an everyday activity (see Exhibit 6–13) • Have patient identify the components of the activity • Have patient arrange the components into a logical order • Have patient estimate the time to complete each component • Move from simple to more complex activities	Percentage correct Percentage correct Time variance between the patient's estimate and the clinician's or caregiver's estimate	

LONG-TERM CLINICAL OBJECTIVE

Patient demonstrates consistent _____ (e.g., reasoning, problem solving) for comprehension and expression of _____ (e.g., legal documents, humor, curriculum-based materials, essays) for _____ (e.g., educational, vocational, avocational) purposes.

Short-Term Clinical Objective	Procedure	Measurement	Comments
Consistent ability to analyze and draw conclusions from contextual cues in a _____ (e.g., picture, written story, video) stimulus	Present a stimulus (e.g., picture depicting a scene, story, the facts of a situation, video); have patient describe the relevant items in the stimulus, determine the relationship of one item to another, and draw conclusions about the stimulus	Number of correct identifications of relevant items versus irrelevant items identified and/or Percentage of conclusions correctly drawn	

continues

Short-Term Clinical Objective	Procedure	Measurement	Comments
Consistent ability to identify and comprehend inconsistencies in _____ (number) _____ (e.g., sentence, paragraph) material	Present sentences, paragraphs, or stories with inconsistencies (e.g., John and James are two men who enjoy many of the same hobbies; people who are racist are usually open minded about diverse cultural and ethnic viewpoints on such issues as affirmative action); have patient identify the inconsistencies	Percentage of inconsistent statements identified out of total possible	Materials for this procedure can come from the patient's own narratives or textual material altered to contain inconsistencies
Consistent comprehension and expression of humor in _____ (number, if appropriate) _____ (e.g., sentence, paragraph, cartoon) material	Present the following materials and have the patient explain the humor: • Jokes • Amusing anecdotes • Puns and double meanings • Cartoons and political satire • Humorists (e.g., Andy Rooney, Erma Bombeck)	Accuracy of rationale for humor	
Consistent expression of a solution to a _____ (e.g., type—see Exhibit 6–14) reasoning task	Present patient with a reasoning task and have patient complete; cue with appropriate strategies for task completion and gradually decrease	Percentage correct and/or Number of cues provided by the clinician and/or Number of self-initiated strategies	
Consistent expression of solution(s) to a problem situation	Present a problem situation (e.g., fires, traffic jams, personal hazards) • Have patient formulate alternate solutions to the problem	Ratio of number of solutions identified by patient to number identified by clinician	
	• Have patient identify consequences of each solution given and then identify the best solution	Number of times patient is able to support responses	

Exhibit 6–11 Outlining

Directions: Read the following paragraphs and identify the main ideas, subtopics, and details. Fill in the appropriate spaces on the outline below.

Last week, 2,000 people watched the Fifteenth Annual College Tennis Tournament at the State University. The Men's Division was won by Jerry Simpson, 22 years of age, from Rockford, Illinois. He defeated 19-year-old Barry Griswald in three sets 6–4, 6–7, 6–3. The match lasted for 3 hours and 22 minutes. Jerry will play in the national competition next month.

Janice Elliot, age 21 years, won the Women's Division. She had an easy victory, 6–1, 6–2, over her long-time opponent, Susan Summers, age 23 years. Summers, who won the championship the last 2 years, graciously complimented Elliot on her victory and wished her luck in the national competition.

Next month's National Tournament will be held in Hilton Head, South Carolina. Over 100 students will participate from around the country. The favorites for the Men's Division are Jim Sampson from California and Dean Davidson from Georgia. The favorites for the Women's Division are Susie Clark from North Carolina and Jennifer Hogan, also from California.

TITLE: THE TENNIS TOURNAMENT

I. _____ (Name of Tournament)
    A. Introduction
        1. _____ (Where It Was Held)
        2. _____ (Size of Audience)
    B. Men's Division Winner
        1. _____ (Name)
        2. _____ (Age)
        3. _____ (Score)
        4. _____ (Name of Opponent)
    C. Women's Division Winner
        1. _____ (Name)
        2. _____ (Age)
        3. _____ (Score)
        4. _____ (Name of Opponent)

II. _____ (Name of Next Tournament)
    A. Introduction
        1. _____ (Where It Will Be Held)
        2. _____ (Number of Participants)
    B. Men's Favorites
        1. _____ (Name and Where From)
        2. _____ (Name and Where From)
    C. Women's Favorites
        1. _____ (Name and Where From)
        2. _____ (Name and Where From)

Exhibit 6–12 Example of Changing Criteria for Prioritizing Information

Example 1: Running errands—prioritize by geographic location
- Hardware store at 600 North Clark Street
- Grocery store at 200 North State Street
- Baker at 780 North Clark Street
- Dry cleaners at 430 North Clark Street
- Drugstore at 333 North State Street

Example 2: Running errands—prioritize by order of importance to prepare for a dinner party
- Hardware store to pick up hammer
- Grocery store to buy meat, vegetables, and fruit
- Bakery to buy dessert
- Dry cleaners to pick up tablecloth and napkins
- Drugstore to buy a new toothbrush

Example 3: Running errands—prioritize so as to run as many errands as possible but with a budgetary constraint of $50
- Hardware store—$7.50
- Grocery store—$45.00
- Bakery—$20.00
- Dry cleaners—$10.00
- Drugstore—$12.00

Source: Reprinted from A.S. Halper, L.R. Cherney, and T.K. Miller, *Clinical Management of Communication Problems in Adults with Traumatic Brain Injury,* © 1991, Aspen Publishers, Inc.

Exhibit 6–13 Examples of Estimating Time To Complete Components of an Activity

CONCRETE OR ROUTINE ACTIVITY: GETTING READY IN THE MORNING

Component	Estimated Time
• Get out of bed and turn off alarm	_____
• Brush teeth	_____
• Shower	_____
• Put on makeup or shave	_____
• Get dressed	_____
• Eat breakfast	_____
Total estimated time	_____

COMPLEX ACTIVITY: CHRISTMAS SHOPPING

Component	Estimated Time
• Make a list of persons (e.g., 2 children, 4 grandchildren, 1 spouse)	_____
• Decide on presents and costs	_____
• Decide on stores	_____
• Buy presents	_____
Total estimated time	_____

Exhibit 6–14 Types of Reasoning Tasks

- Analogies
- Cause and effect
- Determination of valid conclusions
- Drawing morals from a story
- Identification of missing premises
- If–then tasks
- Inferences
- Metaphors, similes, and idioms
- Mindbenders
- Part–whole relationships
- Similarities and differences
- Story completion
- Syllogisms

REFERENCES

1. Damasio AR. *Descartes' Error: Emotion, Reason and the Human Brain.* New York, NY: The Putnam Publishing Group; 1994.
2. Myers PS, Mackisack EL. Right hemisphere syndrome. In: LaPointe LL, ed. *Aphasia and Related Neurogenic Language Disorders.* New York, NY: Thieme Medical Publishers, Inc.; 1990:177–195.
3. Sohlberg MM, Mateer CA. *Attention Processing Training (APT).* Puyallup, Wash: Association for Neuropsychological Research and Development; 1986.
4. Sohlberg MM, Mateer CA. *Attention Processing Training–II (APT–II).* Puyallup, Wash: Association for Neuropsychological Research and Development; 1994.
5. Cherney LR, Halper AS, Drimmer D. Word list recall and recognition by subjects with right hemisphere stroke. *Brain and Language.* 1995; 51:51–53.
6. Sohlberg MM, Mateer CA. *Introduction to Cognitive Rehabilitation: Theory and Practice.* New York, NY: The Guilford Press; 1989.
7. Burke JM, Danick JA, Bemis B, Durgin CJ. A process approach to memory book training for neurological patients. *Brain Inj.* 1994;8:71–81.
8. Burns MS, Halper AS, Mogil SI. Treatment of communication problems in right hemisphere damage. In: Burns MS, Halper AS, Mogil SI, eds. *Clinical Management of Right Hemisphere Dysfunction.* 1st ed. Gaithersburg, Md: Aspen Publishers, Inc.; 1985.
9. Myers PS. Communication disorders associated with right hemisphere brain damage. In: Chapey R, ed. *Language Intervention Strategies in Adult Aphasia.* 3rd ed. Baltimore, Md: Williams & Wilkins; 1994.
10. Sohlberg MM, Perlewitz PG, Johansen A, Schultz L, Hartry A. *Improving Pragmatic Skills in Persons with Head Injury.* Tucson, Ariz: Communication Skill Builders, Inc.; 1992.

Appendix 6–A

Guidelines for Communication Management: Family and Staff

- Treat the individual as an adult
- Strive for communication, not perfection
- Provide reassurance and redirect attention to another task or topic when the individual swears, cries, or displays emotional outburst
- Establish consistent routines to assist the individual's retention and ability to plan the day
- Control the environment to minimize external distractions, thereby helping the patient to focus and maintain attention on the task
- Organize the home environment to aid memory (e.g., keep items in the same place, reduce clutter)
- Post orienting materials like calendars, clocks, and faces of familiar people in a highly visible area
- Rearrange the environment to maximize use of the right visual field if the patient has a left-side neglect
- Compensate for visual impairments through the use of verbal cues
- Draw attention to visual reference points in the room, such as doorways and furniture (e.g., paint the doorknob a bright color or post a large label)
- Avoid rapid movements around the individual
- Establish eye contact prior to giving the patient a message to ensure attention
- Structure and minimize auditory and visual stimulation to permit better attention to the task at hand
- Repeat a statement when uncertain whether the individual was attending
- Be aware that the individual's lack of affect does not necessarily signal disinterest or depression
- Supplement all directions with simple repeated verbal cues, if necessary
- Ask questions during a conversation to ensure that the individual remembers important details and follows topic changes
- Encourage the individual to plan out a task by breaking up the task into a specified number of small steps
- Decrease impulsivity by encouraging the individual to slow down
- Regulate impulsivity by requiring a delay or verbal plan before initiating an activity

Source: Data from A.S. Halper and S. Glista, "Language and Speech Disorders of Neurological Origin in Adults," in *Comprehensive Rehabilitation Nursing*, N. Martin and D. Hicks, eds., © 1981, McGraw Hill; M.S. Burns and A.S. Halper, Language Disorders Associated With Aging, *Topics in Geriatric Rehabilitation*, Vol. 1, No. 4, pp. 15–27, © 1986, Aspen Publishers, Inc.

Appendix 6–B

Publishers of Treatment Materials and Computer Programs

The following is a list of publishers that have a variety of treatment materials and computer programs that are appropriate for use with patients with right hemisphere damage. Specific lists of materials are not included because of the rapid changes in their availability.

Academic Therapy Publications
20 Commercial Boulevard
Novato, CA 94949
(414) 883–3314 or
  (800) 422–7249

Applied Symbolix
16 West Erie Street, Suite 300
Chicago, IL 60610
(312) 787–3772

AGS
4201 Woodland Road
Circle Pines, MN 55014
(800) 328–2560

BrainTrain
727 Twin Ridge Lane
Richmond, VA 23235
(804) 320–0105

Canyonlands Publishing
  Company
10320 W. Indian School Road,
  Suite 6
Phoenix, AZ 85037
(800) 259–2870

Communication Skill Builders
Division of Psychological
  Corporation
555 Academic Court
San Antonio, TX 78204–2498
(800) 228–0752

Critical Thinking Press and
  Software
PO Box 448
Pacific Grove, CA 93950
(408) 375–2455

Edmark Corporation
PO Box 97021
Redmond, WA 98073–9721
(206) 556–8400

IBM Special Needs Systems
Independence Series
  Information Center
1000 NW 51st Street, M/D 5432
Boca Raton, FL 33432
(800) 426–4832

Laureate Learning Systems, Inc.
110 East Spring Street
Winooski, VT 05404
(802) 655–4755

LinguiSystems, Inc.
3100 4th Avenue
East Moline, IL 61244–0747
(800) 776–4332 or
  (309) 755–2300

Parrot Software
PO Box 250755
West Bloomfield, MI
  48325–0755
(800) PARROT 1

PCI Educational Publishing
5221 McCullough Avenue
San Antonio, TX 78212
(800) 594–4263

Pro-Ed, Inc.
8700 Shoal Creek Boulevard
Austin, TX 78758
(512) 451–3246

The Psychological Corporation
555 Academic Court
San Antonio, TX 78204–2498
(800) 232–1223

The Speech Bin, Inc.
1965 Twenty-Fifth Avenue
Vero Beach, FL 32960
(800) 4-SPEECH or
  (407) 770–0007

Thinking Publications
PO Box 163
424 Galloway Street
Eau Claire, WI 54702–0163
(800) 225–4769

Visiting Nurse Service, Inc.
1200 McArthur Drive
Akron, OH 44320
(216) 745–1601 or
  (800) 362–0031

Wayne State University Press
The Leonard N. Simmons
  Building
4809 Woodward Avenue
Detroit, MI 48201–1309
(800) 978–7323

Appendix A

RIC Evaluation of Communication Problems in Right Hemisphere Dysfunction-Revised (RICE-R)

*Anita S. Halper, Leora Reiff Cherney,
Martha S. Burns, and Shelley I. Mogil*

RIC Evaluation of Communication Problems in Right Hemisphere Dysfunction-Revised (RICE-R)

Anita S. Halper
Leora Reiff Cherney
Martha S. Burns
Shelley I. Mogil

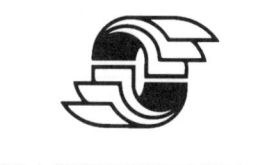

AN ASPEN PUBLICATION

Aspen Publishers, Inc., grants permission for photocopying of this test for limited use within a clinic or other similar organization. This consent does not extend to other kinds of copying, such as copying for general distribution, for creating new collective works, or for resale.

Clinical Management of Right Hemisphere Dysfunction, Second Edition
Copyright © 1996, Aspen Publishers, Inc.

Profile of Severity Ratings (RICE-R)

Name _____   Date _____

Date of Birth _____   Examiner _____

	Normal	Mild	Moderate	Severe
Behavioral Observational Profile	× 23–24	× 19–22	× 14–18	× ≤ 13
Rating Scale of Pragmatic Communication Skills	× 38–40	× 30–37	× 25–29	× ≤ 24
Narrative Discourse—Completeness	× 15–17	× 13–14	× 10–12	× ≤ 9
Visual Scanning and Tracking—Accuracy	× ≤ 5	× 6–16	× 17–70	× ≥ 71
Visual Scanning and Tracking—Rate	× ≤ 210	× 211–390	× 391–549	× ≥ 550
Assessment and Analysis of Writing	× 22–24	× 19–21	× 16–18	× ≤ 15
Metaphorical Language Test	× 20–30	× 17–19	× 13–16	× ≤ 12

Clinical Management of Right Hemisphere Dysfunction, Second Edition
Copyright © 1996, Aspen Publishers, Inc.

Behavioral Observation Profile

INTERVIEW QUESTIONS

Ask each of the following questions in the order given. If the patient is unable to answer a question, then the alternative questions in the parentheses should be asked.

- What is your name? Address?
- Where are you right now? (Are you in the hospital?)
- Why are you here? (Did you have a stroke?)
- When did you first become ill? (When did you have your stroke?)
- How long have you been here in this hospital? (When were you admitted?)
- What is the date today? (What is the day, month, and year?)
- What time is it? (Is it morning or afternoon?)
- What is your occupation?
- What specific problems are you having now? (Can you read and write now? Have you tried since you became ill? Are you having problems identifying your family or friends when they visit? Are you having trouble remembering things? Are you having problems walking?)
- What meals have you eaten today?
- What have you done today before coming here?
- Do you know who I am?
- How long would you say you have been here with me?
- What specific directions would you give a visitor to get from your house to this hospital?

CONVERSATION

Have a five-minute conversation with the patient about a topic of interest (e.g., family or work).

OBSERVATIONS

Observe the patient perform one or more tasks to determine active orientation to place. Examples of tasks follow:

- Find the way from the nursing station to the patient's own room.
- Find the way from the clinician's office to the elevator.
- Find the way from the patient's bed to the bathroom.

Behavioral Observation Profile: Rating Scale

	1	2	3	4
Attention	Inattentive (attentive 0%–30% of the time)	Attentive some of the time (31%–60% of the time)	Usually attentive (61%–90% of the time)	Fully attentive (more than 90% of the time)
Awareness of illness	Denies illness or hemiplegia	Aware of illness and/or some major limitations	Aware of some subtle problems but not all	Fully aware
Orientation to person	Does not recognize family or friends	Recognizes highly familiar people	Recognizes some less familiar people but not all	Oriented
Orientation to place	Unaware of present location	Passive orientation to place but cannot find way around environment	Inconsistently finds way around the environment	Oriented
Orientation to time	Unaware of date, time, season	Aware of gross time periods (e.g., season and month) but not specific times (e.g., date, day of the week)	Aware of specific times and inconsistently monitors the passage of time	Oriented
Memory for daily events	Unable to remember any daily events	Remembers some daily events but not all	Remembers most daily events	Remembers all important daily events

Total Score: _____ / 24

Pragmatic Communication Skills: Rating Scale

NONVERBAL COMMUNICATION

Intonation	1 Flat/monotone or inappropriate	2 Limited or inconsistently appropriate	3 Appropriate intonation most of the time	4 Appropriate
Facial expression	1 Absent or inappropriate	2 Limited or inconsistently appropriate	3 Appropriate facial expression most of the time	4 Appropriate
Eye contact	1 Cannot establish eye contact	2 Needs cues to maintain eye contact	3 Maintains and uses eye contact appropriately most of the time; minimal cues may be needed	4 Appropriate
Gestures and proxemics	1 Absent or inappropriate	2 Limited or inconsistently appropriate	3 Uses gestures and proxemics appropriately most of the time	4 Appropriate

VERBAL COMMUNICATION

Conversation initiation	1 Inappropriate or does not initiate	2 Limited or inconsistently appropriate initiation	3 Initiates conversation appropriately most of the time	4 Appropriate
Turn taking	1 Unaware of turn-taking signals	2 Inconsistently responsive to signals	3 Uses and responds to turn-taking signals appropriately most of the time	4 Appropriate

continues

Topic maintenance	1 Absent or inappropriate topic maintenance (Maintains topic less than 50% of the time)	2 Maintains topic some of the time (50%–75% of the time)	3 Maintains topic most of the time (76%–90% of the time)	4 Maintains topic (more than 90% of the time)
Response length (Circle on scale whether patient produces verbose or short utterances)	1 Responses are verbose or inappropriately short (more than 50% of the time)	2 Responses are inconsistently verbose or inappropriately short (25%–49% of the time)	3 Appropriate response length most of the time (inappropriate only 10%–24% of the time)	4 Appropriate response length (more than 90% of the time)
Presupposition	1 Presupposes too much and/or too little (more than 50% of the time)	2 Presupposes too much and/or too little some of the time (25%–49% of the time)	3 Occasionally presupposes too much and/or too little (10%–24% of the time)	4 Appropriate (more than 90% of the time)
Referencing skills	1 Inappropriate referencing (more than 50% of the time)	2 Inappropriate referencing some of the time (25%–49% of the time)	3 Occasional inappropriate referencing (10%–24% of the time)	4 Appropriate referencing (more than 90% of the time)

Total Score: _____ / 40

Narrative Discourse—Completeness

The following severity levels are based on the Story Retelling-Immediate Subtest of the *Arizona Battery for Communication Disorders of Dementia* by K.A. Bayles, C.K. Tomoeda, Canyonlands Publishing, Inc., Tucson, AZ (1991). This task has a maximum of 17 information units for completeness.

Completeness	Severe ≤ 9 informational units	Moderate 10–12 informational units	Mild 13–14 informational units	Normal ≥ 15 informational units

Visual Scanning and Tracking Instructions

INSTRUCTIONS

    Look at the letter/word on the left (examiner points to target letter/word on the left). Now find and cross out (circle, underline) all the letters/words that are the same as the one on the left.

PRACTICE TEST

A   C   A   G   P   D   A   R   A   U   A

W   W   U   M   N   W   E   I   W   W   P

P   Q   P   R   T   R   Y   S   P   E   P

Clinical Management of Right Hemisphere Dysfunction, Second Edition
Copyright © 1996, Aspen Publishers, Inc.

TASK 1 (22 TARGET LETTERS, 85 TOTAL LETTERS)

```
F  F  R  T  A  F  G  E  F  V  D  F  J  U  I  K  O  F
D  T  R  A  D  E  F  D  S  D  B  G  E  F  D  C  M  N
C  C  R  G  U  T  F  V  C  A  D  F  C  E  O  P  C  H
T  D  E  T  G  V  B  N  M  U  I  T  X  W  T  E  T  H
R  T  G  U  R  D  S  R  X  Z  Q  E  R  V  R  M  O  R
```

___ Number of omissions of target letter
+ ___ Number of nontarget letters selected
= ___ Total number of errors
___ Time in seconds

TASK 2 (39 TARGET LETTERS, 240 TOTAL LETTERS)

a   i e y p e a k z i w q l a k e k a k r h a i w o a n e i a l
     e k f j a i e u w k a o q p w o e i f a k f j r u d j e a q

b   p e o q b d j f u b e j h k r j b h a u b d k e j g y b l s
     r h t j b s j e u g y b d j e h b l a p e i g b h g j t k f

c   e l d k e i c d j e c d y e u q i c f l g k h j c r g t u f
     d j g h t o c l d k g h t c o e j g u c d h e j c d k r h c

d   e i d e l c i d s j e d c j e h g r d c o r i t u y j h k d
     o q p e o t d e c n v b g h d o e i r u y d d a e d j d n g

   Number of omissions of target letter _____
+ Number of nontarget letters selected _____
= Total number of errors _____
   Time in seconds _____

Clinical Management of Right Hemisphere Dysfunction, Second Edition
Copyright © 1996, Aspen Publishers, Inc.
RICE-R:9

TASK 3 (8 TARGET WORDS, 28 TOTAL WORDS)

MATCH   FETCH   HALF   MATH   MATCH   HATCH   MATCH   RETCH

ROUND   SOUND   FOUND   SOUND   HOUND   ROUND   FOUND   ROUND

HARD   HALF   PATH   HARD   HAND   BAND   HARD   CARD

RADIO   RIDE   RODEO   RODEO   RATIO   RADIO   VIDEO   RADIO

   Number of omissions of target word
+ Number of nontarget words selected
= Total number of errors
   Time in seconds

TASK 4 (28 TARGET WORDS, 84 TOTAL WORDS)

the	hte	the	eth	lhe	hen	the	hte	tle	lhe	tch	hte	the	ten	
sit	tis	sit	sil	sid	cit	sit	sit	tis	sid	sil	sit	sid	sit	
let	led	tel	let	ted	det	tel	ted	let	tel	let	ted	let	let	
can	can	cal	lan	can	nan	nac	cac	can	cap	cac	nac	can	lan	
tip	tip	pit	pid	tib	tip	tid	tib	tip	dip	lip	tid	lip	tid	tip
her	her	tel	hen	her	ber	her	hed	her	reh	hen	hep	her	ter	her

Number of omissions of target word
+ Number of nontarget words selected
= Total number of errors
Time in seconds

Clinical Management of Right Hemisphere Dysfunction, Second Edition
Copyright © 1996, Aspen Publishers, Inc.
RICE-R:11

Assessment and Analysis of Writing

ADMINISTRATION

Use lined paper with a left-sided margin for the following writing tasks. Be sure to place the paper directly in front of the patient and not to one side.

1. Have the patient copy the following alphabetically balanced sentence. Use the sentence on a separate page as the stimulus, but have the patient copy it on the lined paper.

    The quick brown fox jumps over the lazy dog

2. Dictate the following words:

    phone
    saw
    ramp
    butter
    chimney
    insist
    little
    annual
    coloring
    January

3. Have the patient write a description of a recent event, or a letter to a friend or family member. If the patient is unable to do this spontaneous writing task, then have the patient write a description of an action picture. Elicit a sample of at least 50 words.

The quick brown fox jumps over the lazy dog

Assessment and Analysis of Writing: Rating Scale

A.

Visuospatial disorganization (lines progressing on a diagonal and superimposed lines)	1 Present	2 Absent
Visuospatial disorganization (superimposed letters)	1 Present	2 Absent
Omission of letters	1 More than three omissions	2 Three or fewer omissions
Perseveration of strokes and/or letters	1 Present	2 Absent
Left-sided neglect (writing begins to right of appropriate left-hand margin)	1 Present	2 Absent

B. Degree of Left-Sided Neglect:
   _____ Score 5: Absent
   _____ Score 4: Less than one-half inch from the margin
   _____ Score 3: One-half inch to two inches from the margin
   _____ Score 2: Two to five inches from the margin
   _____ Score 1: More than five inches from the margin

C. Patients who cannot complete a spontaneous writing sample of at least 50 words are given a rating of 1 (could not do):

Ambiguous sentences (irrelevant/off-topic/redundant)	1 Could not do	2 Present	3 Absent
Run-on sentences (sentences that run into the next sentence with the use of conjunctions or incorrect punctuation)	1 Could not do	2 Present	3 Absent
Incomplete/ungrammatical sentences	1 Could not do	2 Present	3 Absent

Total Score: _____ / 24

Clinical Management of Right Hemisphere Dysfunction, Second Edition
Copyright © 1996, Aspen Publishers, Inc.

Metaphorical Language

Read aloud the following proverbs and idioms, and have patient explain in his/her own words the meaning of each one (e.g., "What would I mean if I said _____?"). Check if response is normal, partially correct, or incorrect to obtain a total score. If qualitative scoring is desired, check appropriate column on the right side of page.

	N 2 POINTS	PC 1 POINT	INC 0 POINTS	PI	LI	R	NR
1. Two heads are better than one							
2. Nothing ventured, nothing gained							
3. Look before you leap							
4. A stitch in time saves nine							
5. He's a chip off the old block							
6. It's raining cats and dogs							
7. Don't beat around the bush							
8. Your name will be mud							
9. It takes two to tango							
10. Save it for a rainy day							
11. He is my right hand							
12. Look down one's nose at							
13. Read between the lines							
14. The apple of my eye							
15. You cannot burn the candle at both ends							

Total Score: _____ / 30

KEY:
N = Normal abstract interpretation
PC = Partially correct
INC = Incorrect

PI = Personal interpretation
LI = Literal interpretation
R = Repeats or nearly repeats the phrase
NR = No response

Appendix B

RIC Evaluation of Communication Problems in Right Hemisphere Dysfunction–Revised (RICE-R)—Administration Manual

*Anita S. Halper, Leora Reiff Cherney,
Martha S. Burns, and Shelley I. Mogil*

Profile of Severity Ratings

The Profile of Severity Ratings is a summary of the raw scores for each subtest. These scores have been assigned to severity ratings according to the guidelines discussed in Chapter 4. An example of a completed profile is provided. The patient's score on each subtest is marked and the points are connected.

Guidelines for determining overall severity are not provided. The clinician should consider the pattern of performance and implications of deficits within each subtest on everyday functioning when determining the overall severity level of the patient.

Profile of Severity Ratings (RICE-R)
Sample

Name _____   Date _____

Date of Birth _____   Examiner _____

	Normal	Mild	Moderate	Severe
Behavioral Observational Profile	×	×	×	×
	23–24	19–22	14–18	13
Rating Scale of Pragmatic Communication Skills	×	×	×	×
	38–40	30–37	25–29	24
Narrative Discourse—Completeness	×	×	×	×
	15–17	13–14	10–12	9
Visual Scanning and Tracking—Accuracy	×	×	×	×
	5	6–16	17–70	71
Visual Scanning and Tracking—Rate	×	×	×	×
	210	211–390	391–549	550
Assessment and Analysis of Writing	×	×	×	×
	22–24	19–21	16–18	15
Metaphorical Language Test	×	×	×	×
	20–30	17–19	13–16	12

Behavioral Observation Profile

ADMINISTRATION

Careful observations of the patient are made during a one-to-one interview followed by a five-minute conversation. The interview questions should be given in the order listed in the test booklet. If the patient is unable to answer a question, then the alternative questions in the parentheses should be asked.

Observe the patient's ability to find the way around the environment (e.g., from the nursing station to patient's own room, from the clinician's office to the elevator, from the patient's bed to the bathroom).

SCORING

The profile is then scored on a scale of 1 to 4 as follows.

Attention

1 = Inattentive; attentive to own name, simple commands, a pointing task, or other stimuli 30% or less of the time

2 = Attentive to stimuli some of the time (31% to 60%) but is easily distracted by extraneous internal or external stimuli, has trouble shifting attention from one task to another, or impulsively responds to stimuli without waiting for completion of the stimulus and assessing all aspects of the situation

3 = Attentive to stimuli most of the time (61% to 90%)

4 = Fully attentive (more than 90% of the time); shifts attention appropriately

Awareness of Illness

1 = Denial of the illness and any obvious impairment such as hemiplegia, hemisensory deficit, or inability to read

2 = Awareness of some problems and/or major limitations; denies other problems, usually less obvious difficulties such as problems with calculation or understanding humor; may express uncertainty about the impairments, such as "They tell me I have muscle weakness," or "I understand I had a stroke"

3 = Awareness of all major limitations; aware of some subtle problems but not all

4 = Full awareness of present limitations relative to premorbid skills; may show anger, depression, or sadness in reaction to the stroke or paralysis, or may have an optimistic outlook

Orientation to Person

1 = Lack of recognition of family or friends

2 = Recognition of highly familiar people

3 = Recognition of some less familiar people; may require contextual and paralinguistic (voice quality) cues to help recognize less familiar people

4 = Easy recognition of family, friends, and less familiar people, although may not remember names

Orientation to Place

1 = Unawareness of present location (e.g., confuses the hospital for a hotel)

2 = Knowledge of basic orienting information about present location (passive orientation), such as hospital; has difficulty moving independently around the environment even in familiar surroundings (active orientation)

3 = Active orientation in familiar environments; difficulty finding way in less familiar surroundings

4 = Passive and active orientation to place

Orientation to Time

1 = Inability to tell time or correctly identify or provide the day, date, year, or season

2 = Awareness of gross time periods such as season, year, and month, but not specific times such as date, day of the week, and time of day

3 = Awareness of specific times (passive orientation), but has difficulty with monitoring the passage of time (active orientation)

4 = Passive and active orientation to time

Memory for Daily Events

1 = Inability to remember any daily events
2 = Memory for some important daily events, but not all
3 = Memory for most daily events
4 = Memory for all daily events

INTERPRETATION

Maximum possible score	24
Normal range	23–24
Severity ratings:	
Mild	19–22
Moderate	14–18
Severe	13 or below

Rating Scale of Pragmatic Communication Skills

The Rating Scale of Pragmatic Communication Skills is divided into two sections:

1. Nonverbal Communication:

   - Intonation: melodic contour and inflectional variations that augment communication

   - Facial expression: variations in facial expression that reflect an individual's general mood and attitude (positive or negative emotions) toward the conversational topic or listener

   - Eye contact: ability to focus initially on a speaker and use appropriate eye contact during conversation; a speaker need not maintain eye contact throughout a dialogue but a listener should maintain eye contact with the speaker to show interest and signal agreement or disagreement

   - Gestures and proxemics: ability to maintain a comfortable distance from the communicative partner and to use spontaneous gestures and changes in body posture to facilitate communication

2. Verbal Communication:

   - Conversational initiation: ability to initiate conversation or new topics

   - Turn taking: ability to alternate conversational turns by responding to and providing nonverbal turn-taking cues such as dropping intonational contour, pausing, and reestablishing eye contact

   - Topic maintenance: ability to maintain a topic over successive utterances or turns

   - Response length: an appropriate response should be long enough to provide new relevant information or to clarify old information that is not presupposed; it should not contain redundant or irrelevant information

   - Presupposition: ability to use shared knowledge between speaker and listener to guide how much information is explicitly verbalized

   - Referencing: appropriate use of pronouns or other referents to refer to previous information or to upcoming information in the dialogue

ADMINISTRATION

Nonverbal and verbal communication skills should be assessed from a dialogue between the clinician and patient in as "natural" a manner as possible. Topics of interest should be discussed to simulate an informal setting rather than a testing situation.

SCORING

The rating scale is scored on a scale of 1 to 4 as follows.

Intonation

- 1 = Flat or monotone without variations appropriate to communicative intent, or consistently inappropriate use of inflectional variations

- 2 = Limited and/or inconsistently appropriate inflectional variations

- 3 = Appropriate intonation most of the time

- 4 = Appropriate inflectional variations that augment communication by signaling turn-taking routines, emphasizing new information, and maintaining interest

Facial Expression

1 = Absent or consistently inappropriate use of facial expressions that draw attention to the speaker in inappropriate ways; does not accurately reflect the emotional content of a message or detracts from communication

2 = Limited and/or inconsistently appropriate use of facial expressions

3 = Appropriate facial expressions most of the time

4 = Appropriate use of facial expression consistent with the communicative intent and attitude toward the conversational topic or listener

Eye Contact

1 = Lack of ability to establish eye contact

2 = Initiation of eye contact at the beginning of a conversation and when there is a change of turn; inability to maintain eye contact without cues

3 = Maintenance and use of eye contact appropriately most of the time; minimal cues may be needed

4 = Appropriate eye contact including using eye contact differently as the role changes from speaker to listener

Gestures and Proxemics

(The patient's physical and motoric limitations should be considered when scoring.)

1 = Absent or consistently inappropriate use of body posture and gestures

2 = Limited and/or inconsistently appropriate use of body posture and gestures

3 = Appropriate gestures and proxemics most of the time

4 = Appropriate use of body posture and gestures to augment verbal expression, to signal turn taking, or to emphasize important points in a conversation

Conversational Initiation

1 = Inappropriate initiation or lack of initiation; speaks only in response to another's questions, provides little or no additional information during a conversation, initiates no topics, or consistently initiates inappropriate topics

2 = Limited or inconsistent initiation of appropriate topics or requests; typically a passive participant in the conversation

3 = Appropriate initiation of conversation most of the time

4 = Appropriate initiation of a variety of speech acts, such as making requests, promises, or reminders; and/or initiates new topics during a conversation

Turn Taking

1 = Unawareness of the listener's signal to change turns and does not use content or cues to guide initiation or end of own turn

2 = Inconsistent use or response to signals to initiate, change, or end turns

3 = Appropriate use or response to turn-taking signals most of the time

4 = Appropriate response to and production of turn-taking signals

Topic Maintenance

1 = Maintenance of topics less than 50% of the time; topics are changed more than one time within a turn, the topic is unclear and/or off-topic comments are made

2 = Maintenance of topic some of the time (50% to 75%)

3 = Maintenance of topic most of the time (76% to 90%)

4 = Maintenance of topic more than 90% of the time; topics change as new information rendered on an old topic raises new questions and inspires comments

Response Length

(Circle on scale whether patient produces verbose or short utterances. Scoring should be considered relative to premorbid style as reported by family members.)

1 = Responses (more than 50%) are too long or too short to provide enough information, so that the intent and content of the utterance is not clear; patient may stray from the topic and provide irrelevant or redundant information.

2 = Responses are too long or too short 25% to 49% of the time.

3 = Responses are appropriate length most of the time (inappropriate only 10% to 24% of the time).

4 = Patient provides appropriate response length (inappropriate less than 10% of the time).

Presupposition

1 = Presupposition of too much and/or too little (50% or more of the time); provides too many or too few details

2 = Presupposition of too much and/or too little some of the time (25% to 49%)

3 = Occasional errors of presupposition; presupposes too much and/or too little (10% to 24% of the time)

4 = Appropriate presupposition (more than 90% of the time); inclusion of necessary information and omission of common knowledge and information that can be inferred from the context

Referencing Skills

1 = Inappropriate referencing; use of vague or improperly placed pronouns or other indefinites to refer to specific bits of information in a conversation more than 50% of the time

2 = Inappropriate referencing some of the time (25% to 49%)

3 = Occasional inappropriate referencing (10% to 24% of the time)

4 = Appropriate use of referents so that the meaning and intent is clear (more than 90% of the time)

INTERPRETATION

Maximum possible score	40
Normal range	38–40
Severity ratings:	
Mild	30–37
Moderate	25–29
Severe	24 or below

Narrative Discourse—Completeness

This task measures the ability to specify all the details in a narrative retelling of a story (completeness).

ADMINISTRATION

Discourse completeness is assessed from the retelling of a short narrative. The Story Retelling Subtest from the *Arizona Battery for Communication Disorders of Dementia*[1] is recommended.

SCORING

Informational units for completeness are scored according to the 17 items listed in the manual for the *Arizona Battery for Communication Disorders of Dementia*.[1]

INTERPRETATION

Severity ratings are assigned as follows:

- SEVERE: Provides 9 or fewer informational units
- MODERATE: Provides 10 to 12 informational units
- MILD: Provides 13 to 14 informational units
- NORMAL: Provides 15 or more informational units

Note: If the Story Retelling-Immediate Subtest of the *Arizona Battery for Communication Disorders of Dementia* is not used, the above scoring is not applicable.

Visual Scanning and Tracking Test

ADMINISTRATION

This subtest contains a practice task, followed by four different scanning tasks including letters and words. The practice task is included to help the patient learn the task. Remind the patient that the target letters change at the beginning of each line.

Place each task midline in front of the patient. It is acceptable for the patient to move the paper to the right or left. Use a stopwatch to time each subtest. Begin timing immediately following your statement "Start this now."

Practice Task

Instruction: Look at the letter on the left (examiner points to target letter on the left). Now find and cross out (circle, underline) all the letters that are the same as the one on the left. Start this now.

Subtest 1: Scanning for Upper-Case Letters

Instruction: Look at the letter on the left (examiner points to target letter on the left). Now find and cross out (circle, underline) all the letters that are the same as the one on the left. Start this now.

Subtest 2: Scanning for Lower-Case Letters

Instruction: Look at the letter on the left (examiner points to target letter on the left). Now find and cross out (circle, underline) all the letters that are the same as the one on the left. Start this now.

Subtest 3: Scanning for Upper-Case Words

Instruction: Look at the word on the left (examiner points to target word on the left). Now find and cross out (circle, underline) all the words that are the same as the one on the left. Start this now.

Subtest 4: Scanning for Lower-Case Words

Instruction: Look at the word on the left (examiner points to target word on the left). Now find and cross out (circle, underline) all the words that are the same as the one on the left. Start this now.

SCORING

Accuracy

Count the number of times the target letter or word is omitted. Also count the number of times a nontarget letter or word is selected. Add the two together for total number of errors.

Rate

Report the time for completion of each subtest in seconds.

INTERPRETATION

Accuracy

Maximum possible errors	437
Normal range	5 or fewer errors
Severity ratings:	
Mild	6–16 errors
Moderate	17–70 errors
Severe	71 or more errors

Rate

Normal range	210 seconds or less
Severity ratings:	
Mild	211–390 seconds
Moderate	391–549 seconds
Severe	550 seconds or more

Assessment and Analysis of Writing

ADMINISTRATION

Use lined paper with a left-sided margin for the following writing tasks. Be sure to place the paper directly in front of the patient and not to one side.

1. Have the patient copy the following alphabetically balanced sentence. Use the sentence on a separate page as the stimulus, but have the patient copy it on the lined paper.

   The quick brown fox jumps over the lazy dog

2. Dictate the following words:

   phone
   saw
   ramp
   butter
   chimney
   insist
   little
   annual
   coloring
   January

3. Have the patient write a description of a recent event, or a letter to a friend or family member. If the patient is unable to do this spontaneous writing task, then have the patient write a description of an action picture, such as the Cookie-Theft Picture from the Boston Diagnostic Aphasia Evaluation.[2] Elicit a sample of at least 50 words.

SCORING

The first five items are scored on a two-part scale that indicates the presence or absence of the following:

- visuospatial disorganization (lines progressing on a diagonal superimposed line)
- visuospatial disorganization (superimposed letters)
- omission of letters
- perseveration of strokes and/or letters
- left-sided neglect (writing that begins to the right of the appropriate left-hand margin)

In addition, degree of left-sided neglect is measured and scored. Measure from the margin to the writing that is furthest away from the margin. Score as follows:

   Score 5 = Absent
   Score 4 = Less than one-half inch from the margin
   Score 3 = One-half inch to two inches from the margin
   Score 2 = Two to five inches from the margin
   Score 1 = More than five inches from the margin

The last three items are scored on a three-part scale. Patients who cannot complete a spontaneous writing sample of at least 50 words receive a rating of 1 (could not do).

- ambiguous sentences (includes irrelevant, off-topic, and/or redundant sentences)
- run-on sentences (sentences that run into the next sentence with the use of conjunctions or incorrect punctuation)
- incomplete sentences or ungrammatical sentences

INTERPRETATION

Maximum possible score	24
Normal range	22–24
Severity ratings:	
Mild	19–21
Moderate	16–18
Severe	15 or below

Metaphorical Language

ADMINISTRATION

Have the patient explain the meaning of each proverb and idiom (e.g., "What would I mean if I said _____?")

SCORING

Check if the response is normal, partially correct, or incorrect. To obtain a quantitative score, score 2 points for normal, 1 point for partially correct, and 0 points for incorrect responses. A maximum of 30 points is possible. Use the following criteria when scoring:

- Normal abstract interpretation (N)—patient gives an appropriate abstract explanation.
- Partially correct (PC)—patient explains the metaphor in an abstract way but with errors or incorrect elaborations.
- Incorrect (INC)—patient gives an incorrect response.

Qualitative scoring of partially correct or incorrect responses may be obtained by checking the following categories:

- Personal interpretation (PI)—patient recognizes the metaphor only as it applies to the patient.
- Literal interpretation (LI)—patient provides concrete interpretation of the metaphor; patient may interpret each word independent of the generalized context.
- Repetition (R)—patient repeats or nearly repeats the phrase; one or two words may be altered.
- No response (NR)—patient provides no attempt to explain meaning.

INTERPRETATION

Maximum possible score	30
Normal range	20–30
High average	28–30
Average	20–27
Severity ratings:	
Mild	17–19
Moderate	13–16
Severe	12 or below

See below for examples of how quantitative and qualitative scores are completed on the test form:

	N (2 POINTS)	PC (1 POINT)	INC (0 POINTS)		PI	LI	R	NR
1. Two heads are better than one								
• Two people working together on a problem can be more effective than one	X							
• Two people working can be better than one		X						
• Like when I had a problem with my car, two mechanics working can fix it better than one		X			X			
• I always do better with help from my wife			X		X			
• A person with two heads is smarter than a person with one head			X			X		

EXAMPLES OF PATIENT RESPONSES AND APPROPRIATE SCORING

1. *Two heads are better than one.*
   - N   Two people working together on a problem can be more effective than one.
   - PC   Two people working can be better than one.
   - PC/PI   Like when I had a problem with my car, two mechanics working can fix it better than one.
   - INC/LI   A person with two heads is smarter than a person with one head.
   - INC/PI   I always do better with help from my wife.

2. *Nothing ventured, nothing gained.*
   - N   If you don't try, you can't succeed.
   - PC   If you try something, you might win, but then you might not.
   - PC/PI   If I don't try to get better, I won't.
   - INC/LI   If you don't venture out of your house, you won't get there.
   - INC/R   Nothing ventured, nothing regained.
   - INC   If there is nothing in the house, you better go to the store.

3. *Look before you leap.*
   - N   Think about the ramifications of your actions before making a move.
   - PC   Before you head out into something, think about what the repercussions might be if you lost, it might be better not to try than to fail.
   - INC/PI   That's my problem, I'm always getting hurt.
   - INC/LI   Watch out before you jump, there may be a big hole.
   - INC   Kangaroos leap very high.

4. *A stitch in time saves nine.*
    - N   If you deal with a problem early before it gets too big, you may be able to solve it and prevent a disaster.
    - PC   It is better to do it now, like the little boy who held his finger in the flood wall and kept the town from going under.
    - PC/PI   If only I had gone to the doctor, I might not be in the hospital because then we would have known about my illness and done something about it.
    - INC/LI   Sew it now and avoid a lot of sewing later.
    - INC/R   A stitch now saves nine.
    - INC   I had nine stitches in my leg.

5. *He's a chip off the old block.*
    - N   The child is just like his father.
    - PC/PI   I look just like my father.
    - INC/LI   The chip is from the same wood as the block.
    - INC/R   He's a piece off the old block.
    - INC   You need wood chips to build a fire.

6. *It's raining cats and dogs.*
    - N   It's raining very hard.
    - PC   It's pouring and that's what most people like when it's very hot.
    - PC/PI   It's like the bad storm that I got caught in and got soaking wet.
    - INC/PI   I like to walk in the rain.
    - INC/LI   It's coming down in animals.

7. *Don't beat around the bush.*
    - N   Don't talk around a subject; get to the point.
    - PC   Don't talk so much or everyone will forget the original question.
    - PC/PI   That's my brother Jack; he's so chatty, you never know what he's getting at.
    - INC/LI   You shouldn't walk around, around, and around the garden.
    - INC/R   Don't beat around the tree.
    - INC   You should watch for thorns on the rose bush.

8. *Your name will be mud.*
    - N   Your reputation will be ruined.
    - PC/PI   That's what I told my kids when they fibbed; everyone will think they are liars even when they tell the truth.
    - INC/LI   Your name badge will get dirty in the mud.
    - INC/R   Your name will be dirt.
    - INC   Clean the mud off your shoes.

9. *It takes two to tango.*
    - N   It takes two people to do certain things.
      OR
      You can't fight without a partner.
    - PC/PI   When my children argue with me, I don't argue back so we can't get into a fight.
    - INC/PI   Now that's the truth, I was always fighting with my brother.
    - INC/LI   It takes two people to dance.
    - INC   Two people are going to the show.

10. *Save it for a rainy day.*
    - N   Save something for when you really need it.
    - PC   Don't spend your money, because one day you'll need it to buy a raincoat for example.
    - INC/LI   Save your money for when it rains or snows.
    - INC/R   Save it for stormy days.
    - INC   You might get wet on a rainy day.

11. *He is my right hand.*
    - N He is my principal assistant and I couldn't do without him.
    - PC/PI That's what my husband is, I can't do without him.
    - INC/PI That's what my husband is.
    - INC/R He is my right arm.
    - INC Most people are right-handed.

12. *Look down one's nose at*
    - N To regard with disapproval
      OR
      To treat disdainfully
    - PC To disapprove of someone so that you don't want to be around them
    - INC/PI That's what my boss sometimes does to me
    - INC/LI To look at the ground
    - INC If you tell lies, your nose will grow longer

13. *Read between the lines.*
    - N To draw certain conclusions that are not apparent on the surface
      OR
      To discern the hidden meaning
    - PC To interpret something
    - INC/PI I have trouble with that since I had my stroke.
    - INC/LI Read within the margins
    - INC To read the book

14. *The apple of my eye*
    - N Extremely dear or much cherished
    - PC/PI My favorite person who lives in New York
    - INC/LI That's the apple I want to eat
    - INC/R The fruit of my eye
    - INC An apple a day keeps the doctor away.

15. *You cannot burn the candle at both ends.*
    - N You cannot exhaust your energies in one direction and yet save them for something else.
      OR
      If you overdo it your health will suffer.
    - PC It's not good to try to do too many things.
    - INC/PI That's what I did before I got sick.
    - INC/LI You can only light the candle on one side.
    - INC You make a wish when you blow out your birthday candles.

REFERENCES

1. Bayles KA, Tomoeda CK. *Arizona Battery for Communication Disorders of Dementia.* Tucson, Ariz: Canyonland Publishing, Inc; 1991.

2. Goodglass H, Kaplan E. *Boston Diagnostic Aphasia Examination.* Philadelphia, Pa: Lea & Febiger; 1983.

Index

A

Acetyltransferase, 10, 11
Achromatopsia, 12
   characteristics of, 12
Acute confusional states, 17
Affect, lack of, 58
Affective auditory agnosia, 15
Affective/emotional aberrations, 14–15
   affective auditory agnosia, 15
   anosognosia, 14
   aprosody, 14–15
   facial recognition defects, 15
Agnosia, environmental agnosia, 12–13
Agraphia, 3
Alexia, 3
Alternating attention, 23
Amnesia, nonverbal amnesia, 16
Analogic reasoning, 25
Anomia, and corpus callosum, 3
Anosodiaphoria, 14
Anosognosia, 14
   characteristics of, 14
Anosognosic overestimation, 14
Aphasia, 3
   and Broca's discovery, 2
Apraxia
   and corpus callosum dysfunction, 3
   and left hemisphere, 2
Aprosody, 14–15
   characteristics of, 14–15
Assessment. *See* Cognitive-communication problems assessment
Attention, 23
   levels of, 23
   and right hemisphere, 5
Attentional disorders, 11–12
   Bookness Program, 61, 65
   and communication problems, 59
   Edgeness Program, 60, 63
   hemispatial neglect, 11–12, 23
   selective attention impairment, 12
   vigilance impairment, 12
Attentional disorders treatment, 59–67
   associative and visual cues, 63
   Attention Process Training Programs, 61
   compensatory attentional tactics, 63
   goals of, 59
   materials for scanning and tracking, 65
   measurement methods, 59–62
   procedures, 59–62
   short-term objectives, 59–62
   tasks for shifting attention, 66
Attention Process Training Programs, 61
Auditory perceptual deficits, types of, 25
Auditory processes
   and left hemisphere, 5
   and right hemisphere, 5
Awareness, types of, 72

B

Behavioral Inattention Test (BIT), 42–43
Behavioral Observation Profile, RICE evaluation, 32, 36, 39
Body image, and left hemisphere, 5
Bogen, Joseph, 4
Bookness Program, 61, 65
Bouillaud, J.B., 2

Brain
  hemispheres, differences between, 9–11
  hemispheric specialization, 1–7
Broca, Paul, 1–2, 9

C

California Verbal Learning Test, 44
Capgras' syndrome, 16–17
  characteristics of, 16–17
Cerebral networks, and cognitive processing, 4
Cognitive-communication impairment, 21–22
Cognitive-communication problems assessment
  Behavioral Inattention Test (BIT), 42–43
  California Verbal Learning Test, 44
  communication guideline management, 97
  Detroit Test of Learning Aptitude, 44–45
  Doors and People, 45–46
  Mini Inventory of Right Brain Injury, 46–47
  RICE evaluation, 31–40
  Right Hemisphere Language Battery, 47–48
  Rivermead Behavioral Memory Test, 49
  Ross Information Processing Assessment, 49–50
  Test of Everyday Attention, 51–52
  treatment materials, listing of, 98
  Verbal and Nonverbal Cancellation Test, 52–53
  Visual Object and Space Perception Battery, 53–54
  Woodcock-Johnson Psychoeducational Battery Revised, 54–55
Cognitive-communication problems treatment
  attentional problems, 59–67
  criteria for participation in treatment, 57–58

  higher-level cognitive processes, 89–95
  memory problems, 72–78
  orientation problems, 79–81
  perceptual deficits, 67–71
  pragmatics problems, 81–89
  therapeutic goals, 58
  treatment team, 58
Cognitive processes
  attention, 23
  interrelationships among, 27
  memory, 23–25
  organization, 25
  orientation, 25–26
  perception, 25
  problem solving, 25
  reasoning, 25
Color vision, loss of, 12
Communication
  discourse production, 26–27
  extralinguistic elements, 26
  language rules, 26
  linguistic elements, 26
  paralinguistic elements, 26
  pragmatics, 26
Communication problems
  cognitive-communication impairment, 21–22
  See also Cognitive-communication problems assessment; Cognitive-communication problems treatment
Compensation strategies, types of, 72
Computed tomography (CT), 4
Computer programs, for treatment, 98
Confusional states, acute, 17
Constructional disability, 13–14
  characteristics of, 13–14
Constructions
  and left hemisphere, 5, 6
  and right hemisphere, 5, 6
Convergent thinking, 25
Conversational discourse, 26–27
Corpus callosum
  dysfunctions and damage to, 3–4
  historical view, 2–3
  split brain studies, 4, 5

D

Damasio, Antonio, 4, 14
Declarative memory, 24
Deductive reasoning, 25
Dejerine, Joseph Jules, 3
Delusions
  Capgras' syndrome, 16–18
  paranoid hallucinatory states, 17
Detroit Test of Learning Aptitude, 44–45
Disconnection syndromes, 2–4
  and corpus callosum, 2–4
Discourse
  conversational discourse, 26–27
  narrative discourse, 26
  procedural discourse, 26
Divergent thinking, 25
Divided attention, 23
Doors and People, 45–46
Dressing disturbances, 14
  characteristics of, 14

E

Edgeness Program, 60, 63
Emotional aberrations. See Affective/emotional aberrations
Emotions, and right hemisphere, 14
Encoding, 23–24
Environmental agnosia, 12–13
  characteristics of, 12–13
Environmental reduplication, 16
Episodic memory, 24

F

Facial expression, defects in, 15
Facial recognition, and left hemisphere, 5, 6
Facial recognition defects, 13, 15
  emotional facial recognition disturbances, 15
  prosopagnosia, 13
Focused attention, 23
Frequency problems, 15–16
Functional MRI (FMRI), 4

G

Galen, 2
Gall, Franz Joseph, 2
Gamma-aminobutyric acid, 10, 11
Geschwind, Norman, 1, 3, 4, 9

H

Hallucinations
    paranoid hallucinatory states, 17
    visual hallucinations, 16
Hemiacalculia, 12
Hemialexia, 12
Hemispatial neglect, 11–12
    characteristics of, 11–12, 23
Hemispheres, anatomical/
    biochemical differences, 9–11
Hemispheric specialization, 1–7
    Broca's discovery, 1–2
    and corpus callosum, 3–4
    disconnection syndromes, 2–4
    history of study of, 1
    left hemisphere, 1–2
    right hemisphere, 4–6

I

Imaging methods, 4
Inductive reasoning, 25

J

Jackson, John Hughlings, 4
Judgment
    meaning of, 25
    social judgment, 25

K

Kaplan, Edith, 3, 4

L

Language
    and left hemisphere, 2, 5, 6
    and right hemisphere, 5

Language rules
    morphology, 26
    phonology, 26
    semantics, 26
Left hemisphere, 1–2
    anatomical characteristics, 10
    biochemistry of, 10
    compared to right hemisphere, 9–11
    functions of, 5, 6
Leipmann, Hugo, 3
Levitsky, Walter, 9
Liepmann, Hugo, 2
Long-term memory, 24
    episodic memory, 24
    semantic memory, 24

M

Magnetic resonance imaging (MRI), 4
Mania, secondary mania, 17
Mathematics
    and left hemisphere, 5
    and right hemisphere, 5, 6
Memory, 23–25
    declarative memory, 24
    encoding, 23–24
    and left hemisphere, 5, 6
    long-term memory, 24
    memorizing process, 23–24
    priming effects, 24
    retrieval, 24
    retrospective memory, 25
    and right hemisphere, 5, 6
    storage, 24
    working memory, 24
Memory disorders, 15–16
    nonverbal amnesia, 16
    recency and frequency problems, 15–16
    reduplicative paramnesia, 16
    visual sequences problems, 16
    working memory disorders, 15
Memory disorders treatment, 72–78
    compensation approach, 72
    functional stimuli for procedures, 73
    measuring, 74–77
    procedures, 74–77

restoration approach, 72
    short-term objectives, 74–77
    tasks performed after designated time period, 78
Metaphorical language test, RICE evaluation, 33, 38, 39–40
Mini Inventory of Right Brain Injury, 46–47
Misoplegia, 14
Morphology, 26
Myers, Ronald, 3

N

Narrative discourse, 26
Neuropsychiatric disorders, 16–17
    acute confusional states, 17
    Capgras' syndrome, 16–17
    paranoid hallucinatory states, 17
    secondary mania, 17
    visual hallucinations, 16
Nonverbal amnesia, 16
    characteristics of, 16
Norepinephrine, 10, 11

O

Organization
    characteristics of, 25
    treatment of problems, 89–91
Orientation, 25–26
    active and passive, 26
    types of, 26
Orientation deficits, characteristics of, 26
Orientation deficits treatment, 79–81
    compensatory strategies, 79
    measurement, 79–81
    organizational devices, 79
    procedures, 79–81
    short-term objectives, 79–81

P

Pallinopsia, 16
Paranoid hallucinatory states, 17
    characteristics of, 17

Perception, nature of, 25
Perceptual deficits
   auditory perceptual deficits, 25
   nature of, 25
   visual perceptual deficits, 25
Perceptual deficits treatment, 67–71
   measurement, 67–70
   procedures, 67–70
   short-term objectives, 67–70
Phonology, 26
Phrenology, 2
Place orientation, 26
Planum temporale, 9
Positron emission tomography (PET), 5
Pragmatics, 26
Pragmatics problems
   extralinguistic problems, 81
   linguistic problems, 81
   paralinguistic problems, 81
Pragmatics problems treatment, 81–89
   family involvement, 81–82
   group setting for, 81
   measurement, 82–88
   procedures, 82–88
   short-term objectives, 82–88
   three phase approach, 81
Praxis, and left hemisphere, 5, 6
Priming effects, 24
Problem solving, 25
   and judgment, 25
   treatment of problems, 91–95
Procedural discourse, 26
Prosody, meaning of, 14–15, 26
Prosopagnosia, 13
   characteristics of, 13

R

Rasch analysis, RICE evaluation, 35, 36, 38
Rating Scale of Pragmatic Communication Skills, RICE evaluation, 32, 36, 39
Reading
   and left hemisphere, 5
   and right hemisphere, 5

Reasoning, 25
   analogic reasoning, 25
   convergent and divergent thinking, 25
   deductive reasoning, 25
   inductive reasoning, 25
   types of reasoning tasks, 95
Reasoning problems, treatment of, 91–95
Recency problems, 15–16
Receptive aprosodia, 15
Reduplicative paramnesia, 16
   characteristics of, 16
Rehabilitation Institute of Chicago Evaluation of Communication Problems in Right Hemisphere Dysfunction (RICE). *See* RICE evaluation
Release hallucinations, 16
Reliability, RICE evaluation, 34–35
Retrieval, memory, 24
Retrospective memory, 25
RICE evaluation
   31–40, Appendix A, Appendix B
   Behavioral Observation Profile, 32, 36, 39
   internal consistency of items, 32–33
   metaphorical language test, 33, 38, 39–40
   Rasch analysis, 35, 36, 38
   Rating Scale of Pragmatic Communication Skills, 32, 36
   reliability, 34–35
   severity levels, determination of, 39–40
   significance testing, 38
   standardization of RICE-R, 33–40
   validity, 35–38
   visual scanning and tracking, 32–33, 39
   writing analysis, 33, 36, 38
Right hemisphere, 4–6
   anatomical characteristics, 10
   biochemistry of, 10
   functions of, 5–6
   compared to left hemisphere, 9–11

Right Hemisphere Language Battery, 47–48
Right hemisphere syndromes
   affective/emotional aberrations, 14–15
   attentional disorders, 11–12
   memory disorders, 15–16
   neuropsychiatric disorders, 16–17
   visuomotor disorders, 13–14
   visuoperceptual disorders, 12–13
Rivermead Behavioral Memory Test, 49
Ross Information Processing Assessment, 49–50

S

Secondary mania, 17
   characteristics of, 17
Selective attention impairment, 12
Selective attention, meaning of, 23
Semantic memory, 24
Semantics, 26
Significance testing, RICE evaluation, 38
Simultanagnosia, 13
   characteristics of, 13
Single photon emission computed tomography (SPECT), 4, 5
Social emotional circuit, 4
Somatophrenia, 14
Speech, and left hemisphere, 5–6
Sperry, Roger, 1, 3, 4
Split brain studies, 4, 5
Spurzheim, Johann Gaspar, 2
Storage, in memory, 24
Sustained attention, 23
Sylvian fissures, 9

T

Test of Everyday Attention, 51–52
Treatment materials, listing of, 98
Treatment. *See* Cognitive-communication problems treatment

V

Validity, RICE evaluation, 35–38
Verbal and Nonverbal Cancellation
  Test, 52–53
Vicq d'Azyr, Felix, 2
Vigilance impairment, 12
Visual disorientation, 13
Visual hallucinations, 16
  characteristics of, 16
  pallinopsia, 16
  release hallucinations, 16
Visual Object and Space
  Perception Battery, 53–54
Visual perceptual deficits, types of,
  25
Visual sequences problems, 16
Visual-tactile processes
  and left hemisphere, 5
  and right hemisphere, 5
Visuomotor disorders, 13–14
  constructional disability,
    13–14
  dressing disturbances, 14
Visuoperceptual disorders,
  12–13
  achromatopsia, 12
  environmental agnosia, 12–13
  facial recognition defects, 13
  prosopagnosia, 13
  simultanagnosia, 13
Vogel, Philip, 4

W

Wernicke, Carl, 2
Willis, Thomas, 2
Woodcock-Johnson
  Psychoeducational Battery
  Revised, 54–55
Working memory, characteristics
  of, 24
Working memory disorders, 15
Writing analysis, RICE
  evaluation, 33, 36, 38
Writing, and left hemisphere, 5

NOTES

NOTES

NOTES

NOTES

NOTES

NOTES

NOTES

NOTES

NOTES

NOTES

NOTES

NOTES

NOTES

NOTES

NOTES

NOTES

NOTES

NOTES

NOTES